Wibke Karin Schulte

D-Dopachrome Tautomerase (D-DT)

Wibke Karin Schulte

D-Dopachrome Tautomerase (D-DT)

Functional Homologue or Cross-Regulator of Macrophage Migration Inhibitory Factor (MIF)?

Südwestdeutscher Verlag für Hochschulschriften

Impressum/Imprint (nur für Deutschland/only for Germany)
Bibliografische Information der Deutschen Nationalbibliothek: Die Deutsche Nationalbibliothek verzeichnet diese Publikation in der Deutschen Nationalbibliografie; detaillierte bibliografische Daten sind im Internet über http://dnb.d-nb.de abrufbar.
Alle in diesem Buch genannten Marken und Produktnamen unterliegen warenzeichen-, marken- oder patentrechtlichem Schutz bzw. sind Warenzeichen oder eingetragene Warenzeichen der jeweiligen Inhaber. Die Wiedergabe von Marken, Produktnamen, Gebrauchsnamen, Handelsnamen, Warenbezeichnungen u.s.w. in diesem Werk berechtigt auch ohne besondere Kennzeichnung nicht zu der Annahme, dass solche Namen im Sinne der Warenzeichen- und Markenschutzgesetzgebung als frei zu betrachten wären und daher von jedermann benutzt werden dürften.

Coverbild: www.ingimage.com

Verlag: Südwestdeutscher Verlag für Hochschulschriften GmbH & Co. KG
Heinrich-Böcking-Str. 6-8, 66121 Saarbrücken, Deutschland
Telefon +49 681 37 20 271-1, Telefax +49 681 37 20 271-0
Email: info@svh-verlag.de

Approved by: Aachen, RWTH, Diss., 2011

Herstellung in Deutschland:
Schaltungsdienst Lange o.H.G., Berlin
Books on Demand GmbH, Norderstedt
Reha GmbH, Saarbrücken
Amazon Distribution GmbH, Leipzig
ISBN: 978-3-8381-3161-0

Imprint (only for USA, GB)
Bibliographic information published by the Deutsche Nationalbibliothek: The Deutsche Nationalbibliothek lists this publication in the Deutsche Nationalbibliografie; detailed bibliographic data are available in the Internet at http://dnb.d-nb.de.
Any brand names and product names mentioned in this book are subject to trademark, brand or patent protection and are trademarks or registered trademarks of their respective holders. The use of brand names, product names, common names, trade names, product descriptions etc. even without a particular marking in this works is in no way to be construed to mean that such names may be regarded as unrestricted in respect of trademark and brand protection legislation and could thus be used by anyone.

Cover image: www.ingimage.com

Publisher: Südwestdeutscher Verlag für Hochschulschriften GmbH & Co. KG
Heinrich-Böcking-Str. 6-8, 66121 Saarbrücken, Germany
Phone +49 681 37 20 271-1, Fax +49 681 37 20 271-0
Email: info@svh-verlag.de

Printed in the U.S.A.
Printed in the U.K. by (see last page)
ISBN: 978-3-8381-3161-0

Copyright © 2012 by the author and Südwestdeutscher Verlag für Hochschulschriften GmbH & Co. KG and licensors
All rights reserved. Saarbrücken 2012

TABLE OF CONTENTS

- A. Abbreviations V
- B. Acknowledgments VII
- C. Publications IX

1 INTRODUCTION 1
1.1 Macrophage Migration Inhibitory Factor 1
1.1.1 MIF – A Historical Overview 1
1.1.2 Molecular Mechanisms of MIF Action 2
1.1.2.1 MIF is a Cytokine 2
1.1.2.2 MIF is a Hormone 3
1.1.2.3 Non-Classical Secretion 4
1.1.2.4 Receptors 4
1.1.2.5 Signaling via ERK-MAPK 5
1.1.2.6 MIF Counteracts Glucocorticoid Effects 6
1.1.2.7 MIF Upregulates TLR4 Expression 6
1.1.2.8 Apoptosis 7
1.1.2.8.1 MIF Suppresses p53 Activity 8
1.1.2.8.2 MIF Signaling via Akt 9
1.1.2.9 MIF Affects Cell Viability and Proliferation 9
1.1.3 MIF in Disease Pathology 10
1.1.3.1 Sepsis 10
1.1.3.1.1 MIF Potentiates Endotoxemia 11
1.1.3.1.2 Serum MIF Levels Increase in Sepsis 12
1.1.3.2 ARDS and Asthma 13
1.1.3.3 Rheumatoid Arthritis 13
1.1.3.4 Atherosclerosis 14
1.1.4 Structure, Enzymatic Activities and Inhibitors 14
1.1.4.1 Three-Dimensional Structure 14
1.1.4.2 Enzymatic Activities 16
1.1.4.3 Small Molecule Inhibitors 17
1.2 *D*-Dopachrome Tautomerase 19
1.2.1 Discovery in Melanoma Cells 19
1.2.2 A Structural Homologue of MIF 19
1.2.3 Tautomerase Activity 20
1.2.4 D-DT in Disease Pathology 21
1.2.4.1 Acute Inflammation 21
1.2.4.2 Neoplasm 22
1.2.4.3 Liver Disease 22

1.3 Specific Aim of this Thesis 23

2 MATERIAL AND METHODS 24
2.1 Cell Lines, Bacteria and Plasmids 24
2.1.1 Cell Lines 24
2.1.2 Bacteria 24
2.1.3 Plasmids 24
2.2 Equipment, Consumables and Chemicals 24
2.2.1 Equipment 24
2.2.2 Consumables 25
2.2.3 Chemicals 25
2.2.4 Multi-Component Systems 26
2.3 Primary and Secondary Antibodies 27
2.3.1 Primary Antibodies 27
2.3.2 Secondary Antibodies 27
2.4 PCR Primers 27
2.5 Media, Buffers and Solutions 27
2.5.1 Media 27
2.5.2 Buffers and Solutions 28
    2.5.2.1 General Buffers 28
    2.5.2.2 Agarose Gel Electrophoresis 28
    2.5.2.3 SDS-PAGE and Western Blot 28
    2.5.2.4 Enzymatic Activity 29
2.6 Molecular Biology Techniques 29
2.6.1 Measurement of DNA Concentration 29
2.6.2 Polymerase Chain Reaction 29
2.6.3 Agarose Gel Electrophoresis 31
2.6.4 Isolation and Purification of DNA from Agarose Gels 32
2.6.5 TOPO Cloning Reaction 32
2.6.6 Heat-shock Transformation of *E. coli* 33
2.6.7 Colony PCR 33
2.6.8 Agarose Gel Electrophoresis of Colony PCR Products 33
2.6.9 Plasmid Isolation 33
2.6.10 Glycerol Cryo Stock of Bacteria 34
2.6.11 DNA Sequencing 34
2.7 Cell Culture Techniques 35
2.7.1 Cultivation and Treatment 35
2.7.2 Cell Thawing 35
2.7.3 Determination of Cell Concentration 35
2.7.4 Cryo Stocks of Cells 36
2.7.5 Transient Transfection 36

    2.7.5.1   Transfection of Fibroblasts by Lipofectamine 2000 36
    2.7.5.2   Transfection of Macrophages by Electroporation............................ 36
  2.7.6 Preparation of Cell Lysates 37
2.8   Functional Assays 37
  2.8.1 Apoptosis Assay 37
  2.8.2 Vitality Assay 39
2.9   Protein Chemistry and Immunology Techniques 40
  2.9.1 Determination of Protein Concentration 40
  2.9.2 SDS-PAGE 40
  2.9.3 Western Blot 41
  2.9.4 Immunodetection 41
    2.9.4.1   Quantification of Band Density 42
  2.9.5 Enzymatic Activity 42
    2.9.5.1   Tautomerase Activity on HPP without Inhibitor 42
    2.9.5.2   Tautomerase Activity on HPP with 4-IPP or ISO-1 42
2.10 *In vivo* Mouse Experiments 43
  2.10.1 LPS Shock 43
  2.10.2 Isolation of Peritoneal Macrophages 43

3   RESULTS 45
3.1   D-DT in Apoptosis 45
  3.1.1 Cloning of D-DT into Mammalian Expression Vectors 45
  3.1.2 D-DT is Overexpressed in Cos-7 Fibroblasts... 46
    3.1.2.1   GFP Transfection Rate of 70% 46
    3.1.2.2   3.8-fold Overexpression of D-DT in Fibroblasts 46
  3.1.3 D-DT is Overexpressed in RAW 264.7 Macrophages 47
    3.1.3.1   GFP Transfection Rate of 35% 47
    3.1.3.2   1.4-fold Overexpression of D-DT in Macrophages 48
  3.1.4 D-DT Does Not Protect from Apoptosis.. 48
3.2   D-DT Enhances Cell Viability 49
3.3   Tautomerization of *p*-Hydroxyphenylpyruvate 50
  3.3.1 Human and Murine D-DT Tautomerase HPP 51
  3.3.2 D-DT is Partially Sensitive to MIF Tautomerase Inhibitors 51
3.4   Neutralization of D-DT Protects Mice from LPS-Shock 54

4   DISCUSSION 55
4.1   D-DT was Overexpressed for Apoptosis Studies 55
  4.1.1 TA Cloning Generates D-DT Plasmid 55
  4.1.2 Lipofectamine 2000 Transfects Fibroblasts 56
  4.1.3 Macrophage Transfection Results from Nucleofection 56

4.2 MIF Acts Anti-Apoptotically..**57**
   4.2.1 D-DT does not Diminish Apoptosis 58
4.3 D-DT Enhances Macrophage Viability..**59**
4.4 MIF and D-DT are Structural Homologues..**61**
   4.4.1 Quantitative Differences in Tautomerase Activity....................................61
   4.4.2 Tautomerase Inhibitors Affect D-DT to Lesser Extent..............................62
   4.4.3 Enzymatic Inhibitors Might Impact Biological Function 62
4.5 Neutralization of D-DT Protects Mice from Endotoxic Shock...................**63**
   4.5.1 D-DT in Human Sepsis is Promising Research Subject 64

5 SUMMARY AND OUTLOOK 66

6 REFERENCES 68

A. Abbreviations

Abbreviations are also defined where they first appear in the text. Amino acids are abbreviated in the three-letter code.

4-IPP	4-iodo-6-phenylpyrimidine
4-OT	4-oxalocrotonate tautomerase
Å	Ångstrom (1 Å = 10^{-10} m)
ABTS	2,2'-azinobis[3-ethylbenzothiazoline-6-sulfonic acid]-diammonium salt
Amp	Ampicillin
bp	Base pair
bpm	Beats per minute
BSA	Bovine serum albumin
CD74	Major histocompatibility complex, class II invariant chain (Ii)
CHMI	5-carboxymethyl-2-hydroxymuconate isomerase
CXXC	Cys-Xaa-Xaa-Cys
D-DT	D-dopachrome tautomerase
DMEM	Dulbecco's modified eagle medium
DMSO	Dimethyl sulfoxide
DNA	Deoxyribonucleic acid
dNTP	Deoxyribonucleotide
DTT	Dithiothreitol
ECM	Extracellular matrix
E. coli	Escherichia coli
EDTA	Ethylenediaminetetraacetic acid
ELISA	Enzyme-linked immunosorbent assay
ERK	Extracellular signal-regulated kinase
EtBr	Ethidium bromide
FBS	Fetal bovine serum
GFP	Green fluorescent protein
hD-DT	Human D-DT
hMIF	Human MIF
HPP	p-Hydroxyphenylpyruvate
HRP	Horseradish peroxidase
IB	Immunoblot
IFN	Interferon
IgG	Immunoglobulin G
IL	Interleukin
ISO-1	(S,R)-3-(4-hydroxyphenyl)-4,5-dihydro-5-isoxazole acetic acid methyl ester
K_d	Dissociation constant
kDa	Kilo-Dalton (1 kDa = 1.6605 x 10^{-21} g)
LB	Luria broth
LPS	Lipopolysaccharide
mD-DT	Murine D-DT
MIF	Macrophage migration inhibitory factor
mMIF	Murine MIF
NaI	Sodium iodide
NRS	Normal rabbit serum
o/n	Overnight

OD	Optical density
PAGE	Polyacrylamide gel electrophoresis
PBS	Phosphate-buffered saline
PCR	Polymerase chain reaction
PVDF	Polyvinylidene fluoride
rD-DT	Recombinant D-DT
rMIF	Recombinant MIF
RNA	Ribonucleic acid
rpm	Revolutions per minute
RT	Room temperature
SDS	Sodium dodecyl sulfate
siRNA	Small interfering RNA
SOC	Super Optimal Broth + glucose
TAE	Tris-acetate-EDTA
TBS	Tris-buffered saline
TE	Tris-EDTA
T_m	Melting temperature
TNF	Tumor necrosis factor
V	Volt

B. Acknowledgments

In the course of my dissertation, I was very fortunate to have the guidance of Univ.-Prof. Dr. rer. nat. Jürgen Bernhagen, Institute of Biochemistry and Molecular Cell Biology at the Rheinisch-Westfälische Technische Hochschule Aachen, and Prof. Richard Bucala, M.D., Ph.D., Department of Internal Medicine Section of Rheumatology at Yale University School of Medicine, New Haven, CT, USA.

Foremost, I gratefully and sincerely thank Univ.-Prof. Dr. rer. nat. Jürgen Bernhagen for being a motivating and committed supervisor throughout the course of my dissertation. His scientific help, support and effort were invaluable for the successful completion of my dissertation. Thank you for enabling me to perform the major part of this thesis abroad at Yale University within the framework of your collaboration with the laboratory of Prof. Richard Bucala, M.D., Ph.D.

I am deeply grateful to Prof. Richard Bucala, M.D., Ph.D., who unhesitatingly gave me the opportunity to work in his laboratory at Yale University. His kind support, guidance and inspiration have provided a great basis for this thesis. He was always accessible and willing to share his immense knowledge of the topic and help me with my research.

I give special thanks to Univ.-Prof. Dr. rer. nat. Lothar Rink for taking time out of his busy schedule to co-evaluate my thesis, and to Univ.-Prof. Dr. med. Andreas Schober for his generous participation on my committee.

I am heartily thankful to all my colleagues in the Bucala and Bernhagen research groups for their help and support. Especially, I wish to thank Dr. Melanie Merk, whose unceasing patience, supportive encouragement, constructive criticism and excellent advice from the day I arrived in New Haven until the last day of writing this thesis, enabled me to develop an understanding of the subject. I thank Dr. Lin Leng for his helpful technical advice and for sharing his wide experience and scientific knowledge during the preparation of this work. I wish to extend my warm thanks to all other lab-mates, in particular Tarah Connolly, Tiffany Sun, Adriana Blakaj, Rita Das, Xin Du, Juan Fan, Marta Piecychna and Bum-Joon Kim, who created a very friendly lab atmosphere and were always helpful with stimulating discussions.

My very special thanks go to my parents, brother, aunt and grandparents for their constant encouragement and support throughout my academic studies and my life.

Lastly, I want to thank all of those who supported me in any aspect during the completion of this thesis and made my stay in New Haven an unforgettable experience in my life. In particular, I want to mention Stephen Kerr, who additionally provided me with valuable linguistic advice in the progress of writing this dissertation.

C. Publications

Parts of my thesis were published in an international peer-reviewed journal:

Merk M, Zierow S, Leng L, Das R, Du X, **Schulte W**, Fan J, Lue H, Chen Y, Xiong H, Chagnon F, Bernhagen J, Lolis E, Mor G, Lesur O, Bucala R. 2011. *The D-dopachrome tautomerase (DDT) gene product is a cytokine and functional homolog of macrophage migration inhibitory factor (MIF)*. Proc Natl Acad Sci U S A 108(34):E577-85.

1 Introduction

1.1 Macrophage Migration Inhibitory Factor

1.1.1 MIF – A Historical Overview

A soluble factor that inhibits the migration of immune cells *in vitro* was mentioned as early as 1932, in reports by Rich and Lewis (1). But the actual discovery of the macrophage migration inhibitory factor (MIF) protein occurred about 30 years later. While developing an assay in 1962 to measure the migration of peritoneal cells in capillary tubes, scientists rediscovered MIF (2). In 1966, David *et al.*, and Bloom and Bennett independently identified MIF as one of the first cytokines (3, 4). The first function attributed to MIF was its inhibitory action on the random migration of macrophages in the delayed-type hypersensitivity reaction (3, 5). Subsequently, MIF was also shown to activate macrophages leading to increased cell surface adhesion and phagocytosis (6). Nevertheless, the molecular mechanisms underlying MIF's functions remained unknown. Several years passed without successful isolation of pure MIF. Samples were contaminated with lipopolysaccharide (LPS), interferon (IFN) γ and interleukin (IL) 4, which possess similar migration inhibitory properties as MIF, making it difficult to distinguish MIF's actions (7-9). A breakthrough came in 1989 when a human T-cell MIF cDNA was first isolated and cloned. The expressed polypeptide had the expected molecular weight of 12.5 kDa (10). In 1993, Bernhagen *et al.* first cloned and purified murine MIF, which they showed was released from anterior pituitary cells in response to bacterial LPS (11). Following the expression of biologically active MIF in *E. coli*, detailed studies on its structure and functions were performed (12). Macrophages, T cells and the pituitary gland were observed to be a major sources of MIF production, releasing the cytokine after treatment with pro-inflammatory stimuli such as LPS, tumor necrosis factor (TNF) α, IFNγ (13), gram-positive exotoxins (toxic shock syndrome toxin-1 (TSST-1) and streptococcal pyrogenic exotoxin A (SPEA)) (14), mycobacterial products (15), malarial pigment (hemozoin) (16), and even after stimulation with low concentrations of anti-inflammatory glucocorticoids (17). In 1999, a MIF knockout mouse was constructed, demonstrating that deletion of the *mif* gene reduces inflammatory responses (18). The discovery of the MIF cell surface receptor CD74 (19) and, later, of the chemokine receptors CXCR2, and CXCR4 (20) helped to further our understanding of the mechanisms for MIF signaling. Reports of an association between high expression *MIF* alleles on the one hand and inflammatory disease susceptibility and severity on the other further emphasized the role of MIF in disease pathology (21-25).

1.1.2 Molecular Mechanisms of MIF Action

1.1.2.1 MIF is a Cytokine

The term cytokine describes a functional class of protein mediators, which are produced in a regulated fashion to affect the activation and differentiation of the immune response. Once released, they usually act in an autocrine or paracrine manner leading to an ensuing activation of the innate (dendritic cell, monocyte/macrophage) or the adaptive (T and B cell) immune response characterized by further production of an array of immunoregulatory cytokines. Cytokines display the cardinal properties of pleiotropism, synergy, antagonism, and redundancy, aggravating the understanding of their precise function in different physiologic and pathologic contexts.

Discovered in the early 1960s as one of the first cytokines to be described, MIF was first considered a T cell cytokine, regulating the activation of T cells induced by mitogenic or antigenic stimuli (14, 26). Monocytes and macrophages that had previously been considered to be the target of MIF action were observed to be a significant source of MIF. Upon pro-inflammatory stimuli, macrophages were reported to produce TNFα and nitric oxide (NO) (13, 27). Subsequently, more cell types, such as eosinophil granulocytes, B cells and mast cells, were identified to be involved in MIF action (28-30). Even gastrointestinal colorectal adenoma cells and prostatic adenocarcinoma cells showed increased MIF levels, suggesting protumorigenic activity of MIF (31, 32). Consistent with its definition as a cytokine, MIF has been shown to exhibit various molecular modes of action relevant to antimicrobial host defense, which are summarized in Figure 1 and further characterized in the subsequent paragraphs.

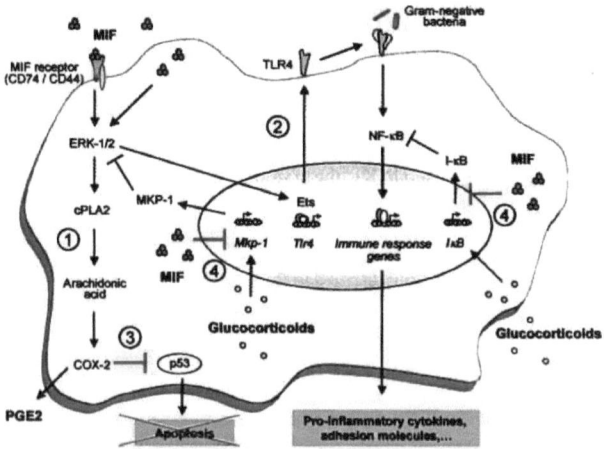

Figure 1: Molecular mechanisms of MIF. MIF binding to the CD74/CD44 receptor complex leads to ERK-1/2 activation, which results in downstream PGE$_2$ production via cPLA$_2$ and COX-2 activation (**1**). Moreover, phosphorylation of ERK-1/2 indirectly upregulates TLR4, the cell surface receptor for gram-negative bacteria, through stabilization of Ets transcription factor (**2**). This results in the upregulation of immune response genes and, thus, production of pro-inflammatory cytokines and adhesion molecules. MIF also protects cells from apoptosis by inhibiting p53 via COX-2 (**3**). The counter-regulation of MIF on the effects of glucocorticoids is summarized in **4**. MIF antagonizes glucocorticoid actions by facilitating the degradation of the NF-κB inhibitor IκB, and also of MKP-1. Abbreviations: ERK-1/2, p44/p42 extracellular signal-regulated kinases; PGE$_2$, prostaglandin E$_2$; cPLA$_2$, cytosolic phospholipase A$_2$; COX-2, cyclooxygenase-2; TLR4, toll-like receptor 4; Ets, E-twenty six; NF-κB, nuclear factor kappa B; IκB, inhibitor of NF-κB kinase; MKP-1, MAPK phosphatase 1. Figure taken from (33).

1.1.2.2 MIF is a Hormone

In 1994, MIF was discovered also to act in a hormone-like fashion. Bernhagen *et al.* identified MIF as a major secreted protein released by anterior pituitary cells in response to septic shock induced by LPS administration (11). MIF expression in corticotrophic and thyrotrophic cells of the anterior pituitary gland and its colocalization in secretory granules with either adrenocorticotrophic hormone (ACTH) or thyroid-stimulating hormone (TSH) further supported MIF's role in the hypothalamic-pituitary-adrenal (HPA) axis (34). Pituitary-derived MIF enters the bloodstream after infectious or stressful stimulation to the organism, leading to an increase of circulating MIF concentrations. A systematic analysis of MIF expression in various organs of the rat showed the release of MIF 6 hours after LPS administration, accompanied by the induction of MIF mRNA and, at 24 hours, the restoration of immunoreactive, intracellular MIF (30). In human serum the physiological MIF serum concentration is between 1 and 15 ng/ml, whereas concentrations up to 350 ng/ml are reached upon inflammatory stimulation (11).

1.1.2.3 Non-Classical Secretion

In contrast to most cytokines, MIF is constitutively expressed and stored in intracellular pools and, therefore, does not require *de novo* protein synthesis before secretion into the extracellular milieu (30). In 1993, Flieger *et al.* demonstrated that MIF secretion occurs via a non-classical export route for protein export, suggesting the involvement of the ATB binding cassette (ABC) A1 transporter (35). More recently, Merk *et al.* identified the Golgi-associated protein p115 as an intracellular binding partner of MIF and provided evidence for the p115-dependent release of MIF from human macrophages (36). It was shown that the small molecule MIF inhibitor 4-IPP targets MIF secretion by influencing the interaction between MIF and p115.

1.1.2.4 Receptors

Cytokines bind to their cell surface receptors and trigger an intracellular signaling cascade. In 2003, CD74 was discovered as the cell surface receptor of MIF (19). CD74 is a 31-41 kDa Type II transmembrane protein and the cell surface form of the Class II-associated invariant chain. Leng *at al.* reported that the cell surface expression of CD74 was required for MIF-dependent ERK-1/2 phosphorylation, prostaglandin E_2 (PGE_2) production and cell proliferation (37). CD74 lacks any obvious signal transduction domain; therefore, the molecular mechanisms of MIF signaling were not evident for some time. In 2007, CD44 was identified as an integral member of the CD74 receptor complex leading to MIF signal transduction. MIF binding to the receptor complex resulted in the serine phosphorylation of CD74 and CD44 at the intracytoplasmic domain (38). Being a widely expressed, polymorphic transmembrane protein with known tyrosine kinase activation properties (39), CD44 then activates members of the Src-family tyrosine kinases, leading to downstream ERK phosphorylation. Both receptors, CD74 and CD44, have been shown to be necessary for MIF protection from apoptosis (38), which further emphasized CD44's role in MIF signaling.

In 2007, Bernhagen et al. identified the chemokine receptors CXCR2 and CXCR4 as non-cognate receptors for MIF (20). MIF competed with cognate ligands and directly bound to CXCR2. CXCR2 and CD74 were shown to co-localize, suggesting a MIF signaling pathway via a CD74/CXCR2 receptor complex. Both receptors were required for MIF-dependent monocyte arrest in atherosclerotic arteries. By activating both CXCR2 and CXCR4, MIF was reported to function as a major regulator of inflammatory cell recruitment and atherogenesis. In 2010, Tarnowski et al. first showed in human rhabdomyosarcoma cells that MIF also stimulates the CXCR7 receptor, resulting in the modulation of tumor metastasis (40).

1.1.2.5 Signaling via ERK-MAPK

In 1999, Mitchell et al. discovered that cell stimulation by MIF let to transient (rapid, within minutes) and sustained (prolonged, for hours) phosphorylation of the p44/p42 extracellular signal-regulated kinases (ERK-1/2) of mitogen-activated protein kinases (MAPK). Activation of ERK-1/2 results in downstream cytoplasmic phospholipase A_2 (cPLA$_2$) activity (37, 41), which is necessary for the production of arachidonic acid. Arachidonic acid acts as the precursor of prostaglandins (*e.g.*, PGE$_2$) and leukotrienes (42, 43), which are expressed in inflammation and mitogenesis (44). cPLA$_2$ is also an important target for the anti-inflammatory action of glucocorticoids (45). Experiments showed that MIF fully diminished glucocorticoid inhibition of cPLA$_2$ activation.

In addition, ERK-1/2 activates several other downstream effector proteins that are involved in the inflammatory response, such as transcription factors (*c-myc*, NF-κB, and Ets) and cytoskeletal proteins mediating membrane activation and phagocytosis (46, 47). Of note, the sustained ERK-1/2 activation is also shared by the stimuli provided by oncogenic mutations in Ras or by integrin co-ligation (48-50), suggesting possible molecular explanations for MIF-induced cell proliferation.

1.1.2.6 MIF Counteracts Glucocorticoid Effects

Surprisingly, Calandra *et al.* demonstrated that macrophage and T cell MIF production was induced by low doses of glucocorticoids (17). Glucocorticoids being powerful anti-inflammatory mediators, these results appeared paradoxical and difficult to reconcile with the pro-inflammatory properties of MIF. However, MIF was subsequently found to override the anti-inflammatory and immunosuppressive effects of glucocorticoids. *In vitro*, MIF reversed glucocorticoid-induced inhibition of pro-inflammatory cytokine synthesis of TNFα, IL-1β, IL-6 and IL-8. Likewise, *in vivo*, MIF overrode the protective effects mediated by glucocorticoids in a mouse model of lethal endotoxemia (17). On a molecular basis, MIF was shown to suppress glucocorticoid-induced expression of anti-inflammatory MAPK phosphatase 1 (MKP-1) (51, 52). MKP-1 is known to inactivate ERK-1/2, p38 and JNK MAPK activities and diminishes cytokine production induced by pro-inflammatory and microbial stimuli (51, 52). MIF also inhibits the steroid-induced upregulation of cytosolic IκB, an inhibitor of the NF-κB pathway (53).

1.1.2.7 MIF Upregulates TLR4 Expression

Sentinel cells of the innate immune system (*e.g.*, monocytes/macrophages, dendritic cells, natural killer cells and granulocytes) possess toll-like receptors (TLR), which are activated by constituents of microbial cell walls or pathogen-specific nucleic acids (54). Upon activation, they initiate the inflammatory host response against infections by stimulating the synthesis and secretion of pro-inflammatory cytokines. In 1999, TLR4 was identified as the signal-transducing molecule of the cell-surface receptor for LPS, a central component of the outer membrane of Gram-negative bacteria (55).

Numerous studies have implicated MIF in host response to LPS, suggesting a molecular basis by which MIF modulates TLR4 expression. Mitchell *et al.* reported that MIF-receptor binding leads to the phosphorylation of ELK-1 (37), which, as a member of the Ets family of transcription factors, is essential for *TLR4* gene transcription (56). MIF-dependent TLR4 upregulation facilitates the detection of endotoxin-containing bacteria and the production of pro-inflammatory cytokines essential for a rapid antimicrobial host response. Accordingly, it was demonstrated that $mif^{-/-}$ macrophages have a reduced expression level of TLR4. The downregulation of TLR4 in *mif*-deficient mice leads to a hyporesponsiveness towards LPS resulting in a reduced production of TNFα, IL-1β, IL-6 and IL-12 (57).

1.1.2.8 Apoptosis

Apoptosis is a physiological cell death program. Its tight regulation is critical for host survival as abnormalities contribute to a variety of human disease (*e.g.*, ischemic damage due to hypertrophy, which facilitates apoptosis in cardiomyocytes, or cancer due to uncontrolled cell proliferation) (58, 59). Cells undergoing apoptosis show specific morphologic characteristics and differ from cells suffering from necrosis, in which the cellular debris can damage the organism. Initiation of apoptosis occurs through multiple independent pathways that derive either from triggering events outside the cell or within the cell (60) (Figure 2). Of note, NO generation in response to a cytokine induced NO-synthase or by NO donors stimulates the expression of the tumor suppressor gene *p53* in macrophages (61). In turn, p53 accumulation in the cytoplasm has a key role in inducing apoptosis, in the maintenance of genomic stability, and in the suppression of transformation and tumorigenesis. Mutations in p53 have been shown to be the most common genetic alteration in human tumors (62).

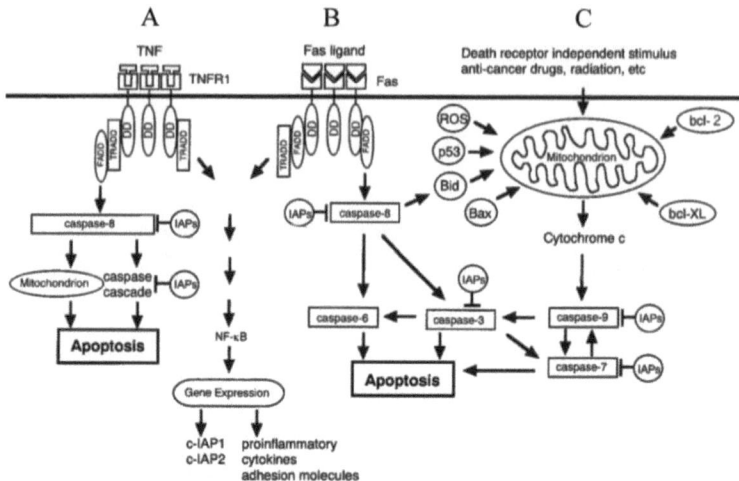

Figure 2: Apoptosis signaling mediated by TNFR, Fas, or mitochondria. Extrinsic initiation of apoptosis by activation of TNFR1 (**A**) or Fas (**B**) results in the recruitment of adaptor proteins (*e.g.*, TRADD, FADD) through interaction with DD. Caspase-8 is activated subsequently. Intrinsic apoptosis (**C**) signaling leads to cytochrome c release from mitochondria, resulting in caspase-9 activation. Interactions with anti-apoptotic (*e.g.*, Bcl-2) or pro-apoptotic (*e.g.*, p53) factors are shown. The activation of caspase-8 or caspase-9 leads to the activation of the caspase-cascade and, thus, to apoptosis. The initiation of the NF-κB signal transduction pathway promotes the transcription of IAPs, as well as pro-inflammatory cytokines. IAPs block different caspases; yet, their precise functions are not fully determined. Abbreviations: TNFR1, TNF receptor-1; TRADD, TNFR1 associated death domain protein; FADD, Fas associated death domain protein; DD, death domain; Bcl-2, B-cell lymphoma 2; IAP, inhibitor of apoptosis. Figure modified from (60).

1.1.2.8.1 MIF Suppresses p53 Activity

When activated (*e.g.*, through LPS-TLR4 interaction), macrophages release NO and other oxide radicals at sites of inflammation (63). Multiple target interactions, *e.g.*, with protein thiol groups, or direct DNA damage with various NO oxidation products serving as the destructive species, have been implicated in NO-mediated cytotoxicity used to kill invading organisms (64). However, NO can also induce apoptosis in macrophages, limiting their inflammatory activities and lifespan, and therefore the inflammatory response over time. In fact, the LPS-induced apoptotic response in macrophages has been shown to require the production of NO, the intracellular accumulation of the tumor suppressor gene product p53, and activation of a caspase-dependent cytolytic pathway (65-68).

In 1999, Hudson *et al.* identified MIF as a negative regulator of p53 activity (62). Three years later, it was demonstrated that MIF sustains macrophage survival by suppressing activation-induced, p53-dependent apoptosis (69). In a model of NO-induced apoptosis, MIF was shown to prevent p53 accumulation in the cytoplasm. The inhibition of p53 activity by MIF requires serial activation of ERK-1/2, cPLA$_2$ and COX-2. Consistent with these findings, LPS-challenge in *mif*-deficient mice results in severely impaired macrophage viability, decreased pro-inflammatory function, and increased apoptotic levels when compared to wild-type macrophages.

1.1.2.8.2 MIF Signaling via Akt

Binding of MIF to the CD74 receptor results in activation of Src kinase and, thus, initiates the phosphoinositide-3-kinase (PI3K)/Akt signaling pathway. Both exogenous recombinant MIF and autocrine MIF action lead to Akt activation and phosphorylation of the pro-apoptotic proteins BAD and Foxo3a (70). BAD phosphorylation impairs its inhibitory action on anti-apoptotic Bcl-2 and protects cells from the deleterious effects of apoptotic stimuli. Moreover, phosphorylation of BAD attenuates death pathway signaling by raising the threshold at which mitochondria release cytochrome c to induce cell death (71).

Another mechanism associated with the ability of Akt to prevent apoptosis is its role in activating NF-κB. Akt stimulates the IκK complex to phosphorylate the NF-κB-inhibitory protein IκB. Thus, with the degradation of IκB, the antiapoptotic transcription factor NF-κB is freed to enter the nucleus where is up-regulates the expression of specific genes involved in immune response, cell survival and proliferation (72). Taken together, these data suggest that MIF's pro-inflammatory actions may be due to its unique ability to affect growth regulation, apoptosis, and cell cycle control of host immune cells.

1.1.2.9 MIF Affects Cell Viability and Proliferation

Apoptosis is crucial for host survival because the timely removal of activated immune cells is an important mechanism for resolving inflammation and immune responses. As MIF suppresses apoptosis, this effect allows for enhanced macrophage survival, increased TNFα, IL-1β, and PGE$_2$ production, and therefore a sustained pro-inflammatory response (69). Mitchell *et al.* showed that endotoxin administration to *mif*$^{-/-}$ mice results in decreased macrophage viability, decreased pro-inflammatory function, and increased apoptosis when compared with wild-type controls (18, 69). Consistent with these findings, inhibition of p53 in endotoxin-treated, MIF-deficient macrophages suppresses enhanced apoptosis and restores pro-inflammatory function.

Mounting evidence suggests that inflammation is closely associated with many types of cancer by promoting an *in vivo* microenvironment which favors tumor growths and metastasis (73). In 1997, Weber *et al.* reported that sustained activation of ERK-1 is required for cyclin D1 expression, which controls the transitions between successive phases of the cell cycle (74). As MIF has been shown to cause both transient and sustained activation of ERK (37), this provides evidence for MIF involvement in promoting cell cycle progression, and thus leading to cell proliferation. However, in 2000, MIF was identified to co-localize and specifically interact with the intracellular protein c-Jun-activation domain-binding protein-1 (JAB1) (75). JAB1 promotes degradation of the cyclin-dependent kinase inhibitor p27^{Kip1}, activates c-Jun amino-terminal kinase (JNK) activity and enhances transcription of AP-1, a transcription factor implicated in cell growth, transformation and cell death. MIF was reported to inhibit these effects and also to antagonize JAB1-dependent cell cycle regulation by increasing p27^{Kip1} expression through its stabilization. Taken together, MIF's effect on macrophage viability and survival provides a mechanism to explain its critical pro-inflammatory action in conditions such as *e.g.*, sepsis or tumorigenesis.

1.1.3 MIF in Disease Pathology

1.1.3.1 Sepsis

Sepsis is an increasingly common cause of morbidity and mortality, particularly in elderly, immunocompromised and critically ill patients. While its mortality rate has decreased during the past decades, it remains high at between 20% to 40% (76). Sepsis and its sequelae have been reported to be the most common cause of death in the nonsurgical intensive care units of the developed world (77). The term sepsis implies a systemic inflammatory response syndrome (SIRS) (Table 1) that arises from infection (78). Severe sepsis is defined as confirmed sepsis with evidence of end-organ dysfunction such as altered mental status, episode of hypotension, elevated creatinine, or disseminated intravascular coagulopathy. It may lead to multiple organ dysfunction syndrome (MODS) involving two or more organ systems or septic shock, both severely critical medical conditions. Septic shock is defined as persistent hypotension despite adequate fluid resuscitation or tissue hypoperfusion manifested by a lactate greater than 4 mg/dl.

More recent studies of the pathophysiology of sepsis revealed a misbalance between pro-inflammatory reactions (designed to kill invading pathogens, but at the same time responsible for tissue damage) and anti-inflammatory responses (designed to limit excessive inflammation, but at the same time making the host more vulnerable for secondary infections) (79).

Table 1: Definition of systemic inflammatory response syndrome (SIRS). SIRS is defined as a systemic inflammatory response to a variety of severe clinical insults resulting in distinct medical conditions. Documented or suspected infection plus conformed SIRS diagnosis criteria is termed sepsis. Table adapted from (80).

Systemic inflammatory response syndrome (SIRS).
Defined by the presence of two or more of the following conditions: (1) Temperature >38 °C or <36 °C (2) Heart rate >90 bpm (3) Respiratory rate >20 bpm (tachypnea), or $PaCO_2$ <32 mmHg (hyperventilation) (4) White blood cell count >12,000 /mm^3, <4,000 /mm^3, or >10 % immature neutrophils ("bands")

1.1.3.1.1 MIF Potentiates Endotoxemia

The administration of lipopolysaccharide (LPS) is generally used to create an *in vitro* or a mouse model of spontaneous sepsis/endotoxemia, which mimics early biochemical, metabolic, hematologic, and cardiovascular septic responses. MIF is rapidly released from immune and pituitary cells after stimulation with LPS, the main virulence factor in the cell wall of gram-negative bacteria (11, 13, 30). Experimental endotoxemia in mice caused a rapid increase in MIF serum levels, peaking 8 – 20 hours after LPS challenge. Concurrent intraperitoneal injection of recombinant MIF protein and LPS resulted in a marked increase in mice mortality. Conversely, pre-treatment with neutralizing anti-MIF antibodies, the small molecule MIF inhibitor

ISO-1 (81), or deletion of the *mif* gene (18) reduced pro-inflammatory cytokine production and increased the survival rate of mice compared to the control group. These results are consistent with models of *E. coli* injection in the peritoneum or cecal ligation and puncture (CLP) (82). An anti-MIF antibody also protected mice from lethal peritonitis, even when treatment was started up to 8 hours after CLP. Likewise, neutralization of MIF activity reduced lung and liver injury and increased survival in models of LPS-induced organ injury, such as acute pancreatitis, or acute hepatic failure (83, 84). Finally, MIF was established as an important mediator of LPS-induced myocardial dysfunction (85). LPS caused MIF release from cardiomyocytes into the systemic circulation, whereas anti-MIF antibodies reversed LPS-induced cardiac dysfunction.

Of note, *Pollak et al.* investigated the role of MIF in susceptibility to bacterial superinfection initiated 48 hours after CLP-induced sublethal peritonitis (86). They reported that neutralization of endogenous MIF increased mortality in response to *Salmonella typhimurium*, *Pseudomonas aeruginosa*, or *Leishmania monocytogenes* superinfection, whereas treatment with recombinant human MIF increased survival. These findings suggest that MIF modulates immune responses with a positive effect on immune-suppressed animals by reenabling them to react adequately to a secondary bacterial challenge.

1.1.3.1.2 Serum MIF Levels Increase in Sepsis

Consistent with the concept established in animal models of septic shock, serum MIF concentrations of patients suffering from sepsis were significantly higher compared to healthy individuals (median MIF concentrations of 111 ng/ml versus 6.3 ng/ml) (87). MIF levels also correlated with the outcome of patients with septic shock as MIF concentrations were measured to be significantly higher in non-survivors than in survivors and remained elevated for several days (88). A recent study suggested MIF as an early predictor for survival in septic patients (89). Thus, were anti-MIF therapeutic strategies to become available in the future, they would have a broad time window of administration and might potentially increase the survival of sepsis.

1.1.3.2 ARDS and Asthma

MIF has been identified as a major regulator in both acute and chronic inflammation. Over time and still to date, MIF involvement in the pathology of an increasing number of diseases has been discovered. Lai *et al.* measured enhanced MIF protein expression in alveolar capillary endothelium and infiltrating macrophages derived from lung tissues of acute respiratory distress syndrome (ARDS) patients in comparison to healthy controls (90). In asthma, a chronic allergic pulmonary disease, similar results were observed. Eosinophils of atopic patients comprised intracellular pools with higher MIF amounts, which were secreted in response to inflammatory stimulation *in vitro*. Alveolar fluids derived from the lungs of stable asthmatic patients contained elevated MIF levels (28). Moreover, neutralization of MIF abrogated the development of airway hyperresponsiveness and airway inflammation in sensitized mice (91). In 2005, genetic analysis of the *MIF* genotype was performed in patients with mild, moderate, or severe asthma (22). Mizue *et al.* observed a significant association between mild asthma and the low expression, 5-CATT *MIF* allele. The human *MIF* gene comprises a CATT-tetranucleotide repeat polymorphism that functionally affects the activity of the *MIF* promoter (24). It is repeated between 5-8 times while a high number of repeats results in an increase in *MIF* promoter activity. The 5-CATT *MIF* promoter polymorphism has also been correlated with low disease severity in rheumatoid arthritis patients.

1.1.3.3 Rheumatoid Arthritis

The first evidence of a role for MIF in rheumatoid arthritis (RA) was provided in 1997 (92). In a mouse model of collagen type-II induced arthritis, neutralization of MIF led to delayed onset and lowered frequency of RA. Treatment with neutralizing anti-MIF antibodies in adjuvant-induced arthritis and antigen-induced arthritis were in accord with these results (93, 94). In RA patients, high amounts of MIF have been detected in synovial fluid and tissues, most notably in fibroblast-like synoviocytes (FLS), macrophages, and T-lymphocytes, which might be the major source of MIF detected in the synovial fluid (95, 96). In 2004, Gregory *et al.* determined that leukocyte migration into the joint space was significantly reduced in *mif*-deficient mice, indicating that MIF is associated with disease activity and preceding structural damage in the joint (97).

1.1.3.4 Atherosclerosis

Furthermore, MIF has been implicated in atherosclerotic plaque development. First evidence for an involvement of MIF in atherogenesis was unveiled in hypercholesterolemic rabbits in 2000. Lin *et al.* reported that MIF was strongly overexpressed in vascular endothelial cells in the early fatty-streak and advanced lesion stages of atherosclerosis, and in monocytes adhering to the endothelial cells (98). Interestingly, this observation was diminished in smooth muscle cells (SMC) in the media of vessels, foam cells and macrophages of advanced plaques, suggesting predominant MIF involvement in early lesion development. In 2002, increased MIF protein expression was reported in human atheroma lesions, which was accompanied by an increase in disease progression. MIF expression in human umbilical vein endothelial cells (HUVEC) was upregulated after stimulation with oxidized low-density lipoprotein (LDL) and macrophages secreted enhanced levels of MIF upon LDL stimulation (99). In a mouse model of spontaneous atherogenesis, treatment with anti-MIF antibody led to a reduction of intimal macrophages, and circulating inflammatory mediators, such as fibrinogen, MIF and IL-6, compared to controls. Accordingly, proteins involved in leukocyte recruitment were reduced upon MIF blockade (100). More recent studies revealed that MIF supports leukocyte recruitment to sites of inflammation by upregulation of intercellular adhesion molecule-1 (ICAM-1) on endothelial cells, and through interaction with the chemokine receptors CXCR2 and CXCR4 (20, 101). Lately, MIF has been proposed to serve as a link between rheumatoid arthritis and atherosclerosis (102), as inflammatory processes in the vessel wall are widely acknowledged to give rise to atherosclerosis (103).

1.1.4 Structure, Enzymatic Activities and Inhibitors

1.1.4.1 Three-Dimensional Structure

Human MIF is a 114-amino-acid non-glycosylated protein of 12,476.3 Da that shows approximately 90% sequence homology in all mammalian species studied so far

(104). Homologues of mammalian MIF have been found not only in mammals but also in both jawless and jawed fish, ticks, the nematodes *C. elegans* and *B. malayi*, cyanobacteria, and plants such as *Arabidopsis thaliana* (105-109).

In 1996, crystallographic studies of human and rat MIF showed that MIF is a homotrimer (110-112). Each monomer contains two antiparallel α-helices and six β-strands; four of these strands form a β-sheet (Figure 3). Performing NMR studies, Mühlhahn *et al.* suggested that the protein could be dimeric in solution (113), whereas cross-linking analysis data even indicated that physiological MIF solutions contain a mixture of monomers, dimers, and trimers (114). The precise determination of the physiological multimerization state of MIF is still not answered to satisfaction.

MIF's three-dimensional oligomeric structure led to the definition of a new protein class named the MIF/tautomerase superfamily. Structurally similar to MIF, other family members are *D*-dopachrome tautomerase (D-DT) and the bacterial enzymes 5-carbodymethyl-2-hydroxymuconate isomerase (CHMI) and 4-oxalocrotonate tautomerase (4-OT) (115).

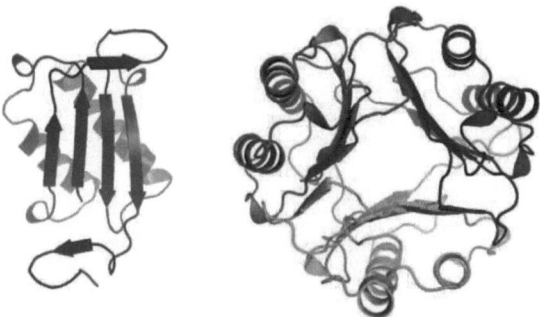

Figure 3: The three-dimensional structure of MIF. *Left:* Human MIF monomer. *Right:* Human MIF trimer. Each monomer contains two antiparallel α-helices that pack against a four-stranded β-sheet. Additionally, each monomer has two β-strands that interact with the β-sheets of adjacent subunits to form the interface between monomers. The three β-sheets are arranged to form a barrel containing a solvent-accessible channel that runs through the center of the protein (110). Structures taken from (116).

1.1.4.2 Enzymatic Activities

To date, two enzymatic activities have been reported for MIF. First, MIF exhibits thiol-protein oxidoreductase (TPOR) activity, which is mediated by a Cys57-Ala-Leu-Cys60 (CALC) sequence motif (117). Although not reconcilable with the static structure of MIF found in crystallographic studies, the cysteines are reported to form a reversible, intramolecular disulfide bridge, which is the catalytic center of MIF (118, 119). Some MIF-mediated immune processes, such as the activation of macrophages, are due to this cysteine-mediated redox mechanism. The CALC motif is structurally sensitive because mutations, especially at Cys60, result in dramatic changes in the folding of MIF. It also lies within the JAB1-binding site (120) that many, but not all, vertebrate homologues possess (106).

Additionally, MIF has been identified as an enzyme that catalyzes the tautomerization of model substrates such as D-dopachrome and p-hydroxyphenylpyruvate (HPP) (121) (Figure 4A and B). To date, the physiological substrate for the tautomerase activity is still unknown. However, the tautomerase activity requires the trimerization of MIF, because the active site is formed between subunits of the trimeric human MIF molecule as described for the substrate HPP (122). HPP interacts with Pro1, Lys32, and Ile64 from one subunit and Tyr95 and Asn97 from an adjacent subunit (Figure 4C). MIF shares this enzymatic activity with all members of the MIF/tautomerase superfamily (D-DT, CHMI, 4-OT). Although there is no sequence homology between MIF, CHMI and 4-OT, the proteins share an N-terminal proline as the catalytic base for the tautomerase activity (122).

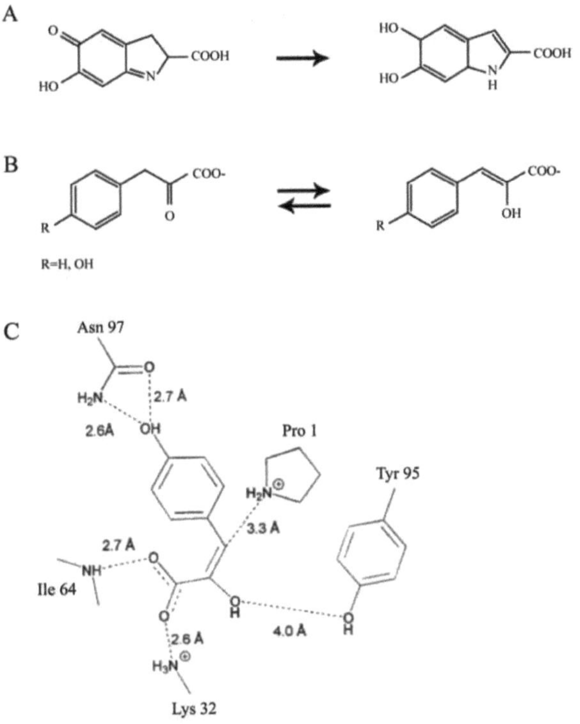

Figure 4: The tautomerase reaction of MIF. A) MIF converts *D*-dopachrome to 5,6-dihydroxyindol-2-carboxylic acid. **B)** MIF also catalyzes the keto-enol isomerization of *p*-hydroxyphenylpyruvate and phenylpyruvate. Structures modified from (116). **C)** Interactions of MIF with the substrate HPP. Structure modified from (122).

1.1.4.3 Small Molecule Inhibitors

Pro-inflammatory function studies of MIF have shown a direct association between the catalytic site surrounding Pro1 and MIF's pro-inflammatory actions. Mutational analysis of the catalytic site around Pro1 led to the conclusion that it is involved in the counter-regulation of glucocorticoids (123), neutrophil priming (124) and the upregulation of metalloproteinases-1 and -3 in rheumatoid arthritis synovial fibroblasts (125). Therefore, it was reasoned that molecules that target this site could be useful to inhibit MIF's actions *in vitro* and *in vivo*. Prototypic small molecules were characterized as catalytic inhibitors of MIF's enzymatic activity by binding to the protein's amino-terminal tautomerase region. Prominent inhibitors are N-acetyl-p-benzo-quinoneimine (NAPQI) (126), (S,R)-3-(4-hydroxyphenyl)-4,5-dihydro-5-isoxazole acetic acid methyl ester (ISO-1) (123), and 4-iodo-6-phenylpyrimidine (4-IPP) (127) (Figure 5).

The reaction between the iminoquinone metabolite of acetaminophen NAPQI and MIF is covalent and produces a NAPQI-modified MIF species with inhibited tautomerase activity, diminished cell-binding ability and decreased immunorecognition (126). ISO-1 binds reversibly to MIF and not only inhibits MIF's tautomerase activity, but also its glucocorticoid counter-regulation activity, MIF-induced production of TNFα, PGE_2 and COX-2 (123), and protects against death in an *in vivo* murine model of endotoxic shock (81). Using computational virtual screening, 4-IPP was identified as a suicide substrate for MIF, causing the covalent modification of Pro1. Functional studies indicated that this compound is approximately 5-10 times more potent than ISO-1 in blocking MIF-dependent catalysis, cell migration and anchorage-independent growth *in vitro* (123). Further differences in the inhibitory potencies of these small molecule inhibitors are evident when comparing the half maximal inhibitory concentration (IC_{50}) determined by the *D*-dopachrome tautomerase assay; ISO-1 has an IC_{50} of ~50 µM, NAPQI of ~40 µM, and 4-IPP of ~5 µM (116).

In 2011, Al-Abed *et al.* reported on the first potential endogenous MIF antagonist, the thyroid hormone thyroxine (T_4) (128). The authors suggested that T_4 might influence MIF-mediated inflammatory responses (*e.g.* survival in mice with severe sepsis) via inhibition of its amino-terminal tautomerase region.

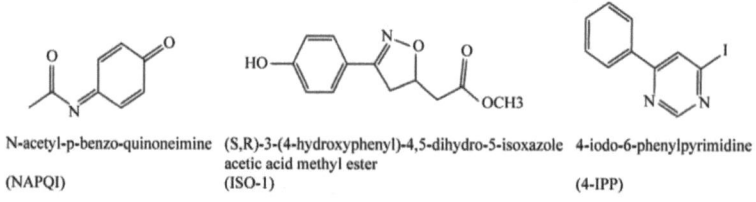

N-acetyl-p-benzo-quinoneimine (S,R)-3-(4-hydroxyphenyl)-4,5-dihydro-5-isoxazole 4-iodo-6-phenylpyrimidine
                                acetic acid methyl ester
(NAPQI)   (ISO-1)   (4-IPP)

Figure 5: Small molecule MIF inhibitors. *Left:* NAPQI. *Middle:* ISO-1. *Right:* 4-IPP. Structures modified from (116).

1.2 D-Dopachrome Tautomerase

1.2.1 Discovery in Melanoma Cells

In 1990, a new protein was purified from mouse melanocytes during an investigation of the regulation of mammalian melanogenesis (129). It was referred to as dopachrome tautomerase according to its tautomerase activity on dopachrome. Aroca et al. reported that dopachrome tautomerase increases the amount of melanin formed from L-tyrosine by melanoma tyrosinase. Subsequently, two membrane-bound L-isomers of dopachrome tautomerase, tyrosinase-related protein-1 and -2 (TRP-1, TRP-2), were defined in melanin forming cells (130, 131). Both enzymes catalyze the isomerization of L-dopachrome to 5,6-dihydroxyindole-2-carboxylic acid (DHICA). In 1993, Odh et al. reported the purification of an enzyme specific for the tautomerization of D-dopachrome, which they named D-dopachrome tautomerase (132). The enzymatic activity of D-DT was described in the liver, kidney, brain, spleen and heart of a male rat as well as in the cytoplasm of human melanoma cells, liver cells, and, later, in blood cells (133).

1.2.2 A Structural Homologue of MIF

D-DT shares very little similarity with any of the L-dopachrome tautomerases. D-DT has been shown to be present in the cytoplasm instead of being membrane-bound (132). Also, the monomer has a low molecular weight (approximately 12 kDa) and a unique amino acid sequence that is not homologues with that of tyrosinase. In 1994, the molecular cloning of D-DT has shown only marginal amino acid sequence homology with either one of the L-dopachrome tautomerases (TRP-1 or TRP-2) (134). However, Merk et al. reported 34% identities in the amino acid sequence between human MIF and D-DT (87). Likewise, their murine homologues share 27% identity and 45% homology (Figure 6). Both proteins are of similar size, about 12 kDa, and Pro1, the catalytic base of the tautomerase activity in MIF, as well as the active site residues Lys32 and Ile64 are conserved in D-DT. Of note, no CALC-motif can be found in D-DT, which is associated with the TPOR activity of MIF (117).

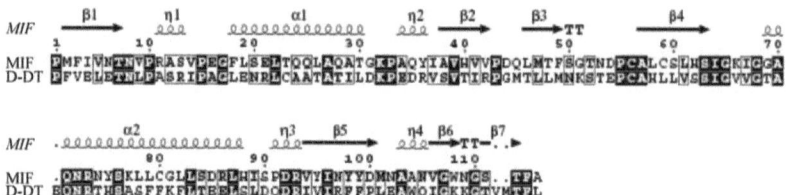

Figure 6: Sequence alignment of murine MIF with murine D-DT. Murine MIF and murine D-DT share 27% sequence identity. A black background marks invariant residues between MIF and D-DT; a box signalizes similar residues. Elements of the secondary structure of murine MIF are shown; α indicates α-helix, whereas β stands for a β-strand of β-sheet, η for a short α-helix and T for turns. Structure modified from (116).

In 1999, Sugimoto *et al.* determined the crystal structure of human D-DT (135) (Figure 7). With respect to the overall three-dimensional (3D) structure of D-DT, it is noteworthy that D-DT shares structural homology with MIF. D-DT's overall homotrimeric folding and its subunit topology are almost identical of human MIF. Each monomer possesses two βαβ motifs and similar trimeric packing by inter-subunit β-sheets compared to MIF.

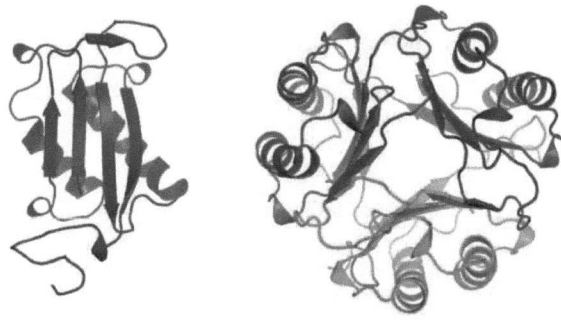

Figure 7: Human *D*-dopachrome tautomerase. Left: human D-DT monomer. Right: human D-DT trimer. Structures taken from (116).

1.2.3 Tautomerase Activity

D-dopachrome and *p*-hydroxyphenylpyruvate have been found to serve as substrates for enzymatic activity of both enzymes, MIF and D-DT (132, 136, 137). In contrast to

MIF, which converts *D*-dopachrome to DHICA, D-DT decarboxylases *D*-dopachrome to 5,6-dihydroxyindole (DHI) (Figure 8).

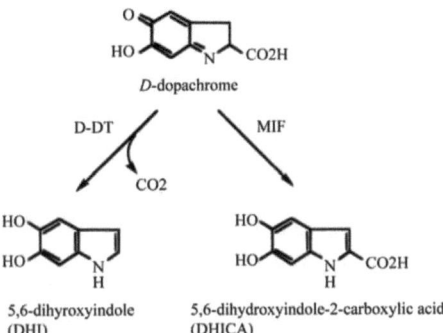

Figure 8: ***D*-dopachrome tautomerization of D-DT and MIF.** Left: D-DT catalyzes *D*-dopachrome to DHI. Right: MIF converts *D*-dopachrome to DHICA. Structures modified from (135).

1.2.4 D-DT in Disease Pathology

To date, there is very little knowledge about the physiological functions and mechanisms of action of D-DT. It is expressed in a large amount in the liver, and to lesser extent in other organs, including the heart, lung and pancreas (138). A first analysis of D-DT expression in murine tissue reveals constitutive and appreciable D-DT levels in several organs with the highest concentration in testis (87).

1.2.4.1 Acute Inflammation

In 2003, Sonesson *et al.* investigated the correlation between UVB-induced skin inflammation and the activity of D-DT in blister fluid (139). In response to UVB light, D-DT activity increased 2-fold, and so did the activity of MIF. These findings provided first evidence of D-DT involvement in inflammation while its co-variation with MIF strengthens this observation. Accordingly, it was reported that D-DT, like MIF, was released from macrophages in response to the pro-inflammatory stimulus LPS (116). The release pattern of both proteins exhibited a bell-shaped curve, that in the case of D-DT peaked at 16 h after LPS stimulation (116). However, cultured macrophages produced 20-fold more MIF than D-DT in response to LPS stimulation.

1.2.4.2 Neoplasm

In 2008, Coleman *et al.* suggested a biological role for D-DT in non-small cell lung carcinomas (NSCLC) (140). The authors showed that the expression of pro-angiogenic factors, such as CXCL8 and vascular endothelial growth factor (VEGF), in NSCLC cells was strongly reliant upon both the individual and cooperative activities of MIF and D-DT. Depletion of MIF and/or D-DT reduced the basal secretion of these two proteins, indicating a tumor-supportive action of D-DT. Tumor-derived growth factors (such as CXCL8 and VEGF) stimulate angiogenesis from surrounding capillaries to support tumor growth and are crucial for tumor progression. MIF and D-DT regulated the CXCL8 transcription via a signaling pathway that appeared to involve JNK, c-JUN and AP-1. Furthermore, the MIF receptor, CD74, was shown to be necessary for MIF- and D-DT-induced JNK activation and CXCL8 expression.

More recently, D-DT was shown to contribute to colorectal cancer disease progression (141). Xin *et al.* observed that D-DT increases COX-2 expression in colorectal adenocarcinoma cell lines through β-catenin stabilization, and activation of c-jun-N-terminal kinase and Jab1/CSN5. As MIF-dependent COX-2 expression has been linked to neoplastic disease progression, these findings suggest a regulatory role for D-DT in cancer pathogenesis.

1.2.4.3 Liver Disease

Proteomic studies of rat liver conducted in 2009 suggested that D-DT is a key protein in liver damage, protection and regeneration (142). A twelve-fold increase in D-DT protein level was measured in rat hepatocytes 24 h after carbon tetrachloride (CCl_4)-induced liver damage compared to control. Protein levels of the antioxidant melanin were also increased in hepatocytes of CCl_4-treated rats. As D-DT has been reported to be involved in the biosynthesis of melanin (132), Hiyoshi *et al.* proposed that increased D-DT levels in response to liver damage could accelerate melanin biosynthesis and therefore protect the liver from oxidative stress. Accordingly, D-DT has been identified as an urinary biomarker of hepatic fibrosis in a rat model of CCl_4-induced hepatic fibrosis (143).

1.3 Specific Aim of this Thesis

The 3D structures of MIF and D-DT are highly conserved. Both proteins possess a tautomerase active site that has its catalytic base in the amino-terminal Pro1. Thus, both proteins belong to the MIF/tautomerase superfamily. However, while the knowledge of MIF's prominent role as a regulator of the innate and adaptive immunity has grown tremendously over the last decades, very little is known about the physiological role of D-DT. As D-DT shows striking structural homology to MIF, it might be suspected that approaches of studying MIF's actions might not be complete without considering D-DT's possible role in disease development. Therefore, detailed functional studies need to be conducted to elucidate whether D-DT exerts similar biological activities to MIF or whether it acts as a cross-regulator or possibly antagonist of MIF. Both scenarios are well documented in immunology.

The aim of this thesis was to investigate D-DT's enzymatic and biological functions to validate previous studies, and to further develop our understanding of D-DT. I first wished to investigate D-DT's influence on cell survival by means of an apoptosis and vitality assay. Second, I wanted to address D-DT's tautomerase activity on the model substrate HPP in comparison to MIF. Also, I planned to probe the effects of catalytic MIF inhibitors on D-DT. Third, the potential effects of an immunoneutralization of D-DT in a murine model of endotoxic shock were to be studied.

2 MATERIAL AND METHODS

2.1 Cell Lines, Bacteria and Plasmids

2.1.1 Cell Lines

Description	Cell type	Morphology
COS-7	African green monkey kidney cells	Fibroblast, adherent
RAW 264.7	Murine ascites leukemia cells	Macrophage/monocyte, adherent

2.1.2 Bacteria

Strain	Genotype	Origin
E. coli TOP10	F⁻ mcrA Δ(mrr-hsdRMS-mcrBC) φ80lacZΔM15 ΔlacX74 recA1 araD139 Δ(ara-leu)7697 galU galK rpsL (Str^R) endA1 nupG	Invitrogen, Carlsbad, CA

2.1.3 Plasmids

Plasmid	Insert	Resistance/Promotor	Origin
pcDNA 3.1	hD-DT	Amp/ T7	this work
pcDNA 3.1	mD-DT	Amp/ T7	this work
pcDNA 3.1	mMIF	Amp/ T7	Bucala lab

2.2 Equipment, Consumables and Chemicals

2.2.1 Equipment

Equipment	Manufacturer
Amaxa nucleofector	Amaxa, Gaithersburg, MD
Analytical balance	Acculab, Columbia, MD
Beckman Alegra6 centrifuge	Beckman, Fullerton, CA
Bright-Line hemacytometer set	Hausser Scientific, Horsham, PA
Centrifuge 5417 R Eppendorf	Eppendorf, Westbury, NY
Centrifuge 5417 R Eppendorf	Eppendorf, Wesseling-Berzdorf, Germany
CO_2 incubator Heracell	Thermo Scientific, Waltham, MA
CO_2 incubator Heracell	Heraeus Instruments, Hanau, Germany
Electrophoresis Power Supply	BioRad, Hercules, CA
Heat block thermo mixer comfort	Eppendorf, Westbury, NY
HERA-Safe sterile bench	Heraeus Instruments, Hanau, Germany
HERA-Safe sterile bench	Thermo Scientific, Waltham, MA
Light microscope	Carl Zeiss, Thornwood, NY
Light microscope Olympus CK40	Olympus Co GmbH, Hamburg, Germany
LSM510 confocal microscope	Carl Zeiss, Thornwood, NY

ND-1000 Spectrophotometer	NanoDrop, Wilmington, DE
NuPAGE/Xcell II Blot Module	Invitrogen, Carlsbad, CA
NuPAGE/Xcell SureLock	Invitrogen, Carlsbad, CA
PTC-100 PCR	BioRad, Hercules, CA
Sorvall Centrifuge	Thermo Scientific, Waltham, MA
SpectraMax Plus	Molecular Devices, Sunnyvale, CA

2.2.2 Consumables

Consumables	Manufacturer
BioMax MR Film	Kodak, Rochester, NY
BioMax MS Film	Kodak, Rochester, NY
Blotting paper	Whatman, Clifton, NJ
Cell culture equipment	BD Falcon, Bedford, MA
	Greiner, Frickenhausen, Germany
Cell scrapers	BD Falcon, Bedford, MA
Centricon	Amicon Bioseparations
Culture Slides	BD Falcon, Bedford, MA
Eppendorf tubes	Eppendorf, Westbury, NY
	Eppendorf GmbH, Wesseling-Berzdorf, Germany
NuPAGE 4-12% Bis-Tris-Gels	Invitrogen, Carlsbad, CA
Polypropylene tubes	BD Falcon, Bedford, MA
PVDF membrane	Millipore, Bedford, MS
Thin wall PCR tubes	BioRad, Hercules, CA

2.2.3 Chemicals

Chemicals	Manufacturer
β-Mercaptoethanol	Sigma, St. Louis, MO
100 bp DNA ladder	Invitrogen, Carlsbad, CA
4-HPP	Sigma, St. Louis, MO
Acetonitrile	J.T. Baker, Phillipsburg, NJ
Agarose	Sigma, St. Louis, MO
Bradford Reagent	BioRad, Hercules, CA
Bromophenol Blue sodium salt	Sigma, St. Louis, MO
BSA	American Bioanalytical, Natick, MA
Dimethylsulfoxide	Sigma, St. Louis, MO
Dithiothreitol (DTT)	Sigma, St. Louis, MO
DMEM	Invitrogen, Carlsbad, CA
	Invitrogen, Eggenstein, Germany
Dry milk powder	BioRad, Hercules, CA
EDTA	American Bioanalytical, Natick, MA
ELC substrate	Pierce, Rockfolrd, IL
FBS	Invitrogen, Carlsbad, CA
	Invitrogen, Eggenstein, Germany
Formaldehyde	American Bioanalytical, Natick, MA
Glycerol	Sigma, St. Louis, MO

Goat serum	Sigma, St. Louis, MO
Imidazole	Sigma, St. Louis, MO
LB Agar Ampicillin-100 Plates	Sigma, St. Louis, MO
Lipofectamine 2000	Invitrogen, Carlsbad, CA
Lipopolysaccharide 0111:B4	Sigma, St. Louis, MO
	Sigma, Munich, Germany
Luria Broth medium	Invitrogen, Carlsbad, CA
Methanol	Fisher Scientific, Pittsburgh, PA
Na_3VO_4	Sigma, St. Louis, MO
NaCl	J.T. Baker, Phillipsburg, NJ
NaF	Sigma, St. Louis, MO
NuPAGE LDS sample buffer	Invitrogen, Carlsbad, CA
NuPAGE SDS running buffer	Invitrogen, Carlsbad, CA
NuPAGE transfer buffer	Invitrogen, Carlsbad, CA
Opti-MEM I Reduced-Serum Medium	Invitrogen, Carlsbad, CA
PCR SuperMix	Invitrogen, Carlsbad, CA
Penicillin/Streptomycin	Invitrogen, Carlsbad, CA
Phosphate buffered saline	Invitrogen, Carlsbad, CA
Protein Free Blocking buffer	Thermo Scientific, Waltham, MA
Protein G Sepharose	Sigma, St. Louis, MO
SeaBlue Plus2	Invitrogen, Carlsbad, CA
SOC medium	Invitrogen, Carlsbad, CA
Sodiumdodecylsulfate	Sigma, St. Louis, MO
Streptavidin-HRP	Promega, Madison, WI
Stripping buffer	Thermo Scientific, Waltham, MA
Superblock	Pierce, Rockfolrd, IL
TAE buffer	Invitrogen, Carlsbad, CA
TMB substrate system	Dako, Carpinteria, CA
Tris	American Bioanalytical, Natick, MA
Triton-X-100	Sigma, St. Louis, MO
Trypsin/EDTA	Invitrogen, Carlsbad, CA
Tween-20	Sigma, St. Louis, MO

2.2.4 Multi-Component Systems

Kits	Manufacturer
Cell Death Detection ELISA [Plus]	Roche, Indianapolis, IN
GeneClean III	MP Biomedicals, Solon, OH
MTT Cell Proliferation Assay Kit	Cayman Chemical, Ann Arbor, MI
Nucleofector Kit V for RAW 264.7	Lonza, Allendale, NJ
pcDNA 3.1/V5-His TOPO TA Expression Kit	Invitrogen, Carlsbad, CA
QIAprep MiniPrep	Qiagen, Valencia, CA

2.3 Primary and Secondary Antibodies

2.3.1 Primary Antibodies

Antigen	Species/Type	Application*	Manufacturer
β-Actin	Mouse IgG$_1$ (monoclonal)	WB	Sigma, St. Louis, MO
D-DT	Rabbit IgG (polyclonal)	WB	Bucala lab
MIF (N20)	Goat IgG (polyclonal)	WB	Santa Cruz Biotechnology, Santa Cruz, CA

*WB: Western blot

2.3.2 Secondary Antibodies

Description*	Species/Type	Application**	Manufacturer
Anti-goat HRP	Donkey	WB	Santa Cruz Biotechnology, Santa Cruz, CA
Anti-mouse HRP	Horse	WB	Cell Signaling, Danvers, MA
Anti-rabbit HRP	Goat	WB	Cell Signaling, Danvers, MA

*HRP: Horseradish peroxidase
**WB: Western blot

2.4 PCR Primers

Description	Sequence
hD-DT-forward	5'-ATGCCGTTCCTGGAGCTG-3'
hD-DT-reverse	5'-GGTCATGACTTTTTTATGA-3'
mD-DT-forward	5'-ATGCCATTCGTTGAGTTG-3'
mD-DT-reverse	5'-GGAACTGTCATGACATTTCTGTGA-3'

2.5 Media, Buffers and Solutions

2.5.1 Media

Complete growth medium for RAW 264.7, COS-7 and mouse peritoneal macrophages	Concentration
DMEM	90%
FBS	10%
Penicillin/streptomycin	1 U/ml

Complete growth medium for COS-7 prior to transfection	Concentration
DMEM	90%
FBS	10%

Quiescent medium for mouse peritoneal macrophages	Concentration
DMEM low glucose	99.9%
FBS	0.1%
Penicillin/streptomycin	1 U/ml

2.5.2 Buffers and Solutions

All buffers were prepared with distilled water, if not stated otherwise.

2.5.2.1 General Buffers

TBS, pH 7.4	Concentration
Tris-HCl, pH 7.4	20 mM
NaCl	150 mM

TBS-T, pH 7.4	Concentration
TBS	(buffer)
Tween-20	0.05%

RIPA	Concentration
Tris-HCl, pH 7.4	50 mM
NaCl	150 mM
EDTA	2 mM
Nonident P-40	1%
Sodium deoxycholate	0.5%
SDS	0.1%
Protease inhibitors complex	1x

2.5.2.2 Agarose Gel Electrophoresis

Gel buffer	Concentration
TAE	(buffer)
EtBr	0.5%

Running buffer	Concentration
TAE	(buffer)

2.5.2.3 SDS-PAGE and Western Blot

Running buffer	Concentration
MES running buffer 20x (NuPAGE)	1x

Transfer buffer	Concentration
Transfer buffer 20x (NuPAGE)	1x
Methanol	10%

Blocking buffer	Concentration
TBS-T	(buffer)
Dry milk powder	5%

Washing buffer	Concentration
TBS-T	(buffer)

2.5.2.4 Enzymatic Activity

HPP buffer, pH 6.0	Concentration
Sodium acetate, 0.05 M	(buffer)
4-HPP	5 mM

HPP buffer was kept dark at room temperature for 24 h in order for HPP to tautomerize into its keto form. It was then stable at 4 °C for two weeks.

Sodium borate buffer, pH 6.2	Concentration
NaOH	(buffer)
Boric acid	0.5 M

2.6 Molecular Biology Techniques

2.6.1 Measurement of DNA Concentration

The concentration and purity of DNA was assessed by photometric analysis using the NanoDrop-1000 Spectrophotometer. The absorption of the nucleotides was measured at OD_{260} and OD_{280}, where 1 OD_{260} value equals 50 µg/ml DNA. The ratio between OD_{260} vs. OD_{280} assesses the purity of the sample with respect to protein contamination. A quotient of 1.8 to 2.0 indicates an uncontaminated sample.

2.6.2 Polymerase Chain Reaction

Polymerase chain reaction (PCR) is used to amplify DNA fragments resulting in thousands to millions of copies of a particular DNA sequence. PCR consists of a

series of 20 to 40 repeated temperature changes called cycles; each cycle typically consists of three discrete temperature steps:

Table 2: Principle of PCR.

Step 1	Denaturation	Heating the reaction to 95°C causes disruption of the hydrogen bonds between complimentary bases, yielding single strands of DNA.
Step 2	Annealing	Lowering the reaction temperature to 50-55°C (~5°C lower than the T_m of the primers used) allows annealing of the primers to the single-stranded DNA template.
Step 3	Elongation	DNA polymerase synthesizes a new DNA strand complementary to the DNA template strand by adding dNTPs in 5' to 3' direction.

Human D-DT (hD-DT) and murine D-DT (mD-DT) cDNA fragments were amplified using *Taq* polymerase, which has its optimum activity temperature at 72°C. The reaction mixture was prepared according to the manufacturer's recommendations. The protocol for amplification included:

hD-DT:

PCR reaction mixture	Amount
PCR SuperMix	45 μl
hD-DT forward primer, 10 μM	1 μl
hD-DT reverse primer, 10 μM	1 μl
hD-DT DNA	2 μl
H$_2$O	1 μl
Total	**50 μl**

Step	Number of cycles	Temperature	Duration
1	1	95 °C	5 min
2	35	95 °C	30 sec
		55 °C	30 sec
		72 °C	1 min
3	1	72 °C	5 min

mD-DT:

PCR reaction mixture	Amount
PCR SuperMix	45 µl
mD-DT forward primer, 10 µM	1 µl
mD-DT reverse primer, 10 µM	1 µl
mD-DT DNA	1 µl
H$_2$O	2 µl
Total	**50 µl**

Step	Number of cycles	Temperature	Duration
1	1	95 °C	5 min
2	35	95 °C	30 sec
		50 °C	30 sec
		72 °C	1 min
3	1	72 °C	5 min

2.6.3 Agarose Gel Electrophoresis

In order to identify and purify DNA after PCR, DNA was separated according to its mass via agarose gel electrophoresis. This was achieved by moving negatively charged nucleic acid molecules through a 1% agarose matrix containing ethidium bromide (EtBr) with an electric field. Smaller molecules moved faster and migrated farther in the gel than bigger ones. EtBr fluoresced under UV light when intercalated into DNA and, thus, visualized DNA bands.

One per cent agarose solution was made in TAE + EtBr buffer and microwaved until the agarose was completely dissolved. After cooling down to about 60 °C, the solution was poured into the gel rack. While continuously cooling down, the agarose polymerized and formed a solid gel. hD-DT and mD-DT PCR products were prepared at a molar ratio of 1:6 in bromophenol blue loading buffer for agarose gel electrophoresis. Fifteen µl of 100 bp DNA ladder and 60 µl of hD-DT and mD-DT PCR samples were loaded into agarose gel slots. After covering the gel completely with TAE, 100 V was applied for 25 min. DNA bands were visualized under UV light.

2.6.4 Isolation and Purification of DNA from Agarose Gels

hD-DT and mD-DT DNA were run on an agarose gel and the desired bands excised from the gel with a razor blade. DNA was eluted using GeneClean® III Kit containing NaI, New Wash and GLASSMILK®. In the presence of NaI, DNA binds to silica beads (GLASSMILK®). After washing off all other proteins, DNA is diluted in TE buffer protecting it from degradation.

The excised DNA/agarose band was weighed and three volumes of NaI solution added (0.1 g DNA/agarose equals 100 µl NaI). The tubes were placed in a 50 °C water bath incubator until the agarose was completely dissolved (approximately 5 min). Fifteen µl of GLASSMILK® suspension was added. The tubes were inverted and incubated at room temperature for 5 min. Then, the DNA/GLASSMILK® solution was centrifuged shortly at 14,000 rpm using a Centrifuge 5417 R (Eppendorf). The supernatant was removed while the pellet contained the DNA/GLASSMILK® complexes. Subsequently, the pellet was washed three times with 750 µl of New Wash. Therefore, the pellet was resuspended in New Wash, centrifuged shortly and the supernatant discarded. Following the washing step, the DNA/GLASSMILK® complexes were eluted into 20 µl of TE buffer by resuspending the pellet. The solution was centrifuged at 14,000 rpm for 1 min. The supernatant containing TE and the eluted DNA was carefully removed and placed in a new tube.

2.6.5 TOPO Cloning Reaction

The TOPO® cloning reaction was set up and incubated at room temperature for 30 min:

TOPO® cloning reaction	Amount
hD-DT / mD-DT DNA	4 µl
Salt Solution	1 µl
TOPO® vector	1 µl
Total	**6 µl**

2.6.6 Heat-shock Transformation of *E. coli*

After thawing an aliquot of competent cells on ice, bacteria were incubated with 2 µl of hD-DT / mD-DT TOPO® cloning reagent for 30 min on ice prior to transformation. Heat-shock transformation occurred via incubation for 30 s at 42 °C. Subsequently, bacteria were kept on ice for two minutes and incubated at 37 °C in 250 µl of SOC medium for 1 h. Bacteria were plated on LB-agar plates containing 100 µg/ml ampicillin and incubated o/n at 37 °C.

2.6.7 Colony PCR

In order to determine whether the hD-DT / mD-DT DNA was inserted into the TOPO® vector, colony PCR was performed. The components of the colony PCR reaction mixture are listed below, whereas the colony PCR protocol was performed according to the PCR amplification protocol (paragraph 2.6.2).

Colony PCR reaction mixture	Amount
PCR SuperMix	45 µl
hD-DT / mD-DT forward primer, 10 µM	1 µl
hD-DT / mD-DT reverse primer, 10 µM	1 µl
Half of an *E. coli* colony	~ 1 µl
H_2O	2 µl
Total	**50 µl**

2.6.8 Agarose Gel Electrophoresis of Colony PCR Products

The agarose gel electrophoresis of colony PCR products was performed according to the agarose gel electrophoresis protocol (paragraph 2.6.3).

2.6.9 Plasmid Isolation

E. coli colonies, which have been proven to contain hD-DT or mD-DT DNA in their transformed vectors, were grown at 37 °C o/n in 5 ml of LB medium subjoined with carbenicillin at a final concentration of 50 µg/ml. The next day, plasmids were isolated with the QIAprep MiniPrep according to the manufacturer's recommendations. Four ml of LB medium containing bacteria were centrifuged at 3,000 rpm at 4 °C for 10 min (Beckman Alegra6 centrifuge). The supernatant was removed, the pelleted bacterial cells resuspended in 250 µl of buffer P1 and transferred into a microcentrifuge tube. Then, 250 µl of buffer P2 and 350 µl of buffer N3 were added and thoroughly mixed by inverting the tube a few times. The mixture was centrifuged at 13,000 rpm at room temperature for 10 min and the supernatant pipetted to the QIAprep spin column. Subsequently, it was centrifuged at 10,000 rpm at room temperature for 1 min. Washing the QIAprep spin column with 750 µl of buffer PE containing ethanol was followed by DNA elution. To do so, the QIAprep spin column was placed in a clean microcentrifuge tube, 50 µl of H_2O added and incubated at room temperature for 1 min. After centrifuging at 13,000 rpm at room temperature for 1 min, the flow-through contained the isolated hD-DT / mD-DT plasmid.

2.6.10 Glycerol Cryo Stock of Bacteria

One ml of LB medium containing hD-DT or mD-DT transformed *E. coli* bacteria were pipetted into cryo tubes. Subsequently, 150 µl of 100% Glycerol was added. Tubes were vortexed and stored at - 80 °C for further use.

2.6.11 DNA Sequencing

DNA sequencing, which was conducted by the W. M. Keck Foundation Biotechnology Resource Laboratory (Yale University), confirmed successful cloning. The protocol for sample submission included:

DNA sequencing	Concentration	Amount
hD-DT / mD-DT plasmid	~ 300 ng/µl	2 µl
T7 primer	50 ng/µl	2 µl
H_2O		14 µl
Total		**18 µl**

2.7 Cell Culture Techniques

2.7.1 Cultivation and Treatment

All cell culture work was performed in BL-2-approved laminar flow hoods. For cultivation, cells were kept in a humidified atmosphere at 37 °C with 5% CO_2. All media and solution were sterile and endotoxin free.

Adherent cells were passaged at a confluence of 70 – 80%. Cells were washed twice with PBS. RAW 264.7 macrophages were detached from culture flasks using a cell scraper, whereas Trypsin/EDTA was used for COS-7 fibroblasts. Cells were re-plated in fresh medium at a confluence of 10%.

2.7.2 Cell Thawing

An aliquot of cells was removed from liquid nitrogen (-196 °C) and immediately immersed into 37 °C water bath until the medium was completely liquid. Nine ml of pre-warmed complete growth medium was added in order to reduce the toxicity of the dimethyl sulfoxide (DMSO) contained in the cell solution. Subsequently, cells were centrifuged at 1,000 rpm for 5 min (Beckman Alegra6 centrifuge), resuspended in pre-warmed complete growth medium, transferred into cell culture flasks and incubated at 37 °C.

2.7.3 Determination of Cell Concentration

Cells were washed with PBS, detached from cell culture flasks, and suspended in the desired medium. An aliquot of 10 µl was placed on the hemacytometer chamber and the number of cells determined by counting. The formula for calculating the cell concentration in the mixture included:

Table 3: Formula for determination of cell concentration.

$N = n * 10^4$
(N = number of cells per ml; n = cell number counted in one hemacytometer square)

2.7.4 Cryo Stocks of Cells

A maximal confluence of 90% of cells plated in complete growth medium was desired prior to cryo stock preparation. Cells were detached from flasks and suspended in cryo medium at a concentration of 1×10^6/ml. Cryo medium consisted of FBS and 5% DMSO. Aliquots of 1 ml were pipetted into cryo tubes and subsequently cooled down. Cryo stocks were stored in liquid nitrogen.

2.7.5 Transient Transfection

Depending on the cell type, different methods were employed for transfection. Successful transfection was determined by GFP detection under a fluorescent microscope 48 h later.

2.7.5.1 Transfection of Fibroblasts by Lipofectamine 2000

The cationic, lipid-based transfection reagent Lipofectamine 2000 was used to transfect plasmid DNA into *in vitro* cell cultures of COS-7 fibroblasts. Lipofectamine treatment altered the cellular plasma membrane, allowing nucleic acids to cross into the cytoplasm.

One day before transfection, COS-7 fibroblasts were plated in complete growth medium without antibiotics at a concentration of 1×10^5/ml. Thus, a cell confluence of 90-95% was achieved at the time of transfection. Then, 0.8 µg of plasmid DNA (either GFP, mMIF or mD-DT plasmid) and 2 µl Lipofectamine 2000 were diluted separately in 50 µl of Opti-MEM I Reduced-Serum Medium. After incubating at room temperature for 5 min, the diluted plasmid DNA was combined with the diluted Lipofectamine 2000. This was succeeded by incubation at room temperature for 20 min. Subsequently, 100 µl of plasmid DNA / Lipofectamine 2000 complexes were added to each well containing COS-7 cells and medium. Cells were cultured at 37 ° between 24 h and 48 h after transfection.

2.7.5.2 Transfection of Macrophages by Electroporation

RAW 264.7 macrophages were transfected with plasmid DNA by Amaxa electroporation. Electroporation significantly increases the permeability of the cell plasma membrane by applying an external electrical field, allowing cellular introduction of DNA, which would never passively diffuse across the hydrophobic bilayer core.

Preparation of RAW 264.7 macrophages for transfection included the following steps: cultivation of cells in complete growth medium, washing of cells with PBS, dislodging cells from culture flasks by scraping, counting cells, transferring aliquots of $2x10^6$ cells into 15 ml Falcon tubes, centrifuging cells at 1000 rpm at 20 °C for 10 min. Next, the cell pellet was resuspended in 100 µl room temperature nucleofector solution V. Two µg plasmid DNA (either GFP, mMIF or mD-DT plasmid) was added and sample transferred into an Amaxa certified cuvette. The Nucleofector program D-032 was selected for electroporation. To avoid damage of the cells, samples were removed from the cuvette immediately after electroporation had finished. After electroporation, transfected macrophages were transferred into 6-well cell culture plates containing 2 ml pre-warmed complete growth medium per well and incubated at 37 °C for 48 h.

2.7.6 Preparation of Cell Lysates

Preparation of cell lysates for Western blot analysis included the following steps: washing of cells with ice cold PBS, lysis of cells by incubation in 200 µl RIPA buffer containing protease and phosphatase inhibitors for 30 min at 4 °C, removal of genomic DNA and cell debris by centrifugation at 14,000 rpm at 4 °C for 10 min.

2.8 Functional Assays

2.8.1 Apoptosis Assay

Roche's Cell Death Detection ELISA^{PLUS} was used for the detection of D-DT's effect on macrophage apoptosis. This assay is based on a quantitative sandwich-enzyme-immunoassay-principle, which quantifies histone-complexed DNA fragments (mono- and oligonucleosomes) in the cytoplasmic fraction of cell lysates (Figure 9).

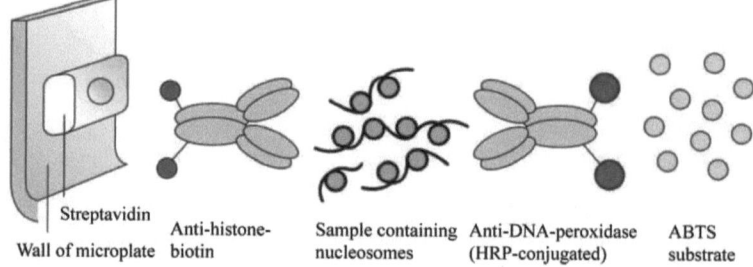

Figure 9: Principle of the Cell Death Detection ELISA^{PLUS}. The sample (*e.g.*, cell lysate) is placed into a streptavidin-coated microplate. A anti-histone-biotin antibody binds to the histone-component of the nucleosomes in the sample and simultaneously captures the immunocomplex to the streptavidin-coated microplate via its biotinylation. Additionally, the anti-DNA-peroxidase antibody reacts with the DNA-component of the nucleosomes. Following removal of unbound components by a washing step, the amount of nucleosomes is quantitatively determined by the peroxidase retained in the immunocomplex. The amount of peroxidase is determined photometrically with ABTS as substrate. Abbreviations: HRP, Horseradish peroxidase. Figure modified from Roche.

RAW 264.7 macrophages were transfected with GFP, mMIF or mD-DT plasmid. Right after transfection, cells were plated in a 96-well cell culture plate at a cell density of 1×10^5/ well in complete growth medium and incubated at 37 °C for 48 h. A working solution of 100 mM sodium nitroprusside (SNP) was prepared and 1 µl pipetted into each well of the 96-well cell culture plate containing macrophages and complete growth medium. Thus, a final SNP concentration of 1 mM was generated. Cells were incubated at 37 °C for another 4 h and the ELISA assay was performed. Cell medium (containing necrotic cell DNA which had leaked through the cell membrane during incubation) was removed and 200 µl lysis buffer added to each well. Following an incubation time of 30 min at room temperature, cell lysates were centrifuged at 1000 rpm for 10 min. An aliquot of 20 µl from the supernatant (cytoplasmic fraction) was transferred into the streptavidin-coated well of a microplate. After preparing the immunoreagent according to the manufacturer's recommendations and adding 80 µl to each well, the microplate was covered with an adhesive cover foil and incubated under gentle shaking for 2 h at room temperature. During this process, the nucleosomes in the supernatant of the cell lysate were bound with two monoclonal antibodies, anti-histone (biotin-labeled) and anti-DNA (HRP-conjugated). Antibody-nucleosome complexes were bound to the microplate by the streptavidin. Subsequently, the solution was removed thoroughly by trapping and the microplate washed three times with 250 μl incubation buffer per well in order to remove cell components that were not immunoreactive. The samples were incubated with 100 μl of HRP substrate (ABTS solution) on a plate shaker until the color development was sufficient for a photometric analysis (approximately 10 min). Then, 100 μl ABTS stop solution was added to each well in the following. The amount of colored product (and thus, of immobilized antibody-histone complexes) was determined spectrophotometrically at 405 nm.

2.8.2 Vitality Assay

Cayman's MTT Proliferation Assay Kit is a colorimetric assay system applicable for studying cell viability in an *in vitro* model. In this assay, cells take up MTT, a yellow tetrazole, due to its net positive charge and the plasma membrane potential. Intracellular MTT is reduced into an insoluble, purple formazan product by NAD(P)H-oxidoreductases in the mitochondria of viable cells. After cell lysis and solubilization of these purple crystals into a colored solution, the samples are read on a microplate reader. The amount of color produced is directly proportional to the number of viable cells.

Mouse peritoneal macrophages were collected and seeded in a 96-well microplate containing complete growth medium at a cell density of 1×10^5 /well. After an incubation at 37 °C for approximately 5-6 hours, macrophages had become adherent. Cell medium was then changed to DMEM low glucose, low FBS in order to quiescent macrophages for further investigation and incubated overnight. The next day, cells were washed three times with PBS. Quiescent cell medium containing either recombinant MIF, D-DT, or both MIF and D-DT was added at a final concentration of 50 ng/ml. Subsequently, macrophages were incubated at 37 °C for 2 h. Ten μl of MTT reagent was added, the microplate gently shaken, and the cells again incubated for 4 h. After incubation, the formazan produced in the cells appeared as dark crystals in the bottom of the wells. The culture medium was carefully aspirated from each well to prevent disruption of the cell monolayer. Subsequently, 100 μl of crystal dissolving solution was added to each well, dissolving the formazan crystals and producing a purple solution. The absorbance to each sample was measured at 570 nm using a microplate reader.

2.9 Protein Chemistry and Immunology Techniques

2.9.1 Determination of Protein Concentration

The concentration of protein in solution was measured by a spectroscopic analytical procedure according to Bradford (144). The previously red coomassie reagent changes and stabilizes into coomassie blue after binding of hydrophobic amino acids of protein. Bound coomassie is blue, with an absorption spectrum maximum at 595 nm, while the unbound forms are green or red. The increase of absorbance at 595 nm is proportional to the amount of bound dye, and thus to the amount (concentration) of protein present in the sample.

After diluting the Bradford reagent 1:5 in water, samples were diluted 1:1000 in Bradford solution. A BSA standard with BSA concentrations from 0 µg/ml to 20 µg/ml was performed accordingly. After incubation for 5 min at room temperature, the absorbance was measured at 595 nm. The concentration of the samples was calculated by interpolation from a BSA standard curve (BSA concentration over OD_{595} values).

2.9.2 SDS-PAGE

Proteins were separated according to their size (and therefore, molecular weight) in an externally applied electric field. The NuPAGE system was employed using Bis-Tris 4-12% polyacrylamide gradient gels.

Samples were boiled in sodium dodecylsulfate (SDS) sample loading buffer for 10 min. In this progress, the negatively charged detergent SDS denatures native proteins by binding to polypeptides in a constant weight ratio of 1.4 g per 1 g of polypeptide. Thus after treatment, polypeptides get a linear structure possessing a uniform negative charge density due to SDS. Besides SDS, the reducing agent DTT denatures the proteins further by reducing disulfide linkages. After denaturation, 20 µl of sample was pipetted into the gel slot and separated at 160 V in NuPAGE/XCell SureLock chambers for 10 min followed by 200 V for 50 min. MES running buffer was used for small molecular weight proteins in the range of 3-50 kDa. As voltage was applied, the polypeptides moved through the gel matrix at different speeds toward the anode determined by their molecular weight. Smaller proteins traveled farther down the gel, while larger ones remained closer to the point or origin. One lane was reserved for SeaBlue Plus2 marker, a mixture of proteins having defined molecular weights and stained so as to form visible, colored bands.

2.9.3 Western Blot

Proteins separated in SDS-PAGE were transferred to a methanol-activated PVDF membrane using the XCell II Blot Module. Proteins maintained the organization they had within the gel, but were available for detection. Therefore, SDS-PAGE gel and PVDF membrane were stacked in the blot module surrounded by filter papers and pads, which were soaked in transfer buffer in order to keep the components moist. The inner chamber was also filled with transfer buffer, while ice and ice cold water was poured in the outer chamber. The blotting process was run at 40 V for 60 – 90 min.

2.9.4 Immunodetection

Following Western blotting, the unspecific binding sites on the PVDF membrane were blocked by incubating it in 10 ml blocking buffer for 2 h. The primary antibody was diluted at a ratio of 1:1000 in blocking buffer and the membrane was incubated with primary antibody solution either for 2 h at room temperature or overnight at 4 °C. Previous to incubating the blotting membrane with the HRP-coupled secondary antibody, it was washed 3 times. The secondary antibody was diluted in blocking solution at 1:5000 and incubated with the membrane for 1 h. After washing the membrane, proteins were visualized by detecting the chemiluminescence emitted after addition of the ECL substrate. If the membrane was re-probed, the membrane was incubated in stripping buffer for at least 30 min at room temperature. After thoroughly washing the membrane, immunoblotting procedure was repeated.

2.9.4.1 Quantification of Band Density

To quantify the bands obtained via Western blot analysis, ImageJ software analysis (http://rsb.info.nih.gov/ij/) was applied. The area under the curve (AUC) of the specific signal was corrected for the AUC of the loading control. The value for the 'GFP' condition was set as 1, and other conditions were recalculated correspondingly to allow ratio comparisons.

2.9.5 Enzymatic Activity

p-Hydroxyphenylpyruvate (HPP) served as a substrate for the tautomerase activity of human MIF, human D-DT and murine D-DT. Therefore, 64 µM dilutions of each protein in PBS were prepared.

2.9.5.1 Tautomerase Activity on HPP without Inhibitor

The tautomerase reaction was set up as followed and activity of the protein was measured by the difference in absorbance at 305 nm in a spectrophotometer over the course of 3 min:

Tautomerase reaction	Amount
Sodium borate buffer	452 µl
H_2O	77 µl
Protein	1 µl
HPP	17 µl

2.9.5.2 Tautomerase Activity on HPP with 4-IPP or ISO-1

4-IPP and ISO-1 were diluted in DMSO to a final concentration of 100 mM. For their administration in the tautomerase assay, the stock solution was diluted further according to the following tables:

Protein, concentration	4-IPP, concentration	Protein: inhibitor ratio
64 µM	64 µM	1:1
64 µM	320 µM	1:5
64 µM	640 µM	1:10
64 µM	6.4 mM	1:100

Protein, concentration	ISO-1, concentration	Protein: inhibitor ratio
64 µM	6.4 mM	1:100
64 µM	64 mM	1:1000
64 µM	640 mM	1:10,000

Protein and inhibitor were combined and incubated at room temperature for 10 min. Subsequently, the tautomerase reaction was set up and remaining activity of the protein was measured photometrically:

Tautomerase reaction	Amount
Sodium borate buffer	452 µl
H_2O	77 µl
Protein/inhibitor solution	1 µl
HPP	17 µl

2.10 *In vivo* Mouse Experiments

All experiments were performed in compliance with the guidelines of the Yale University Institutional Animal Care and Use Committee.

2.10.1 LPS Shock

LPS shock experiments were performed with 6 - 8 week old female BALB/c mice. First, 200 µl of anti-mD-DT serum or normal rabbit serum (NRS) were injected intraperitoneally 2 h prior to LPS injection. Then, 20 mg/kg LPS (0111:B4) was applied for survival experiments. Subsequently, mice were observed for the following 2 weeks.

2.10.2 Isolation of Peritoneal Macrophages

Peritoneal macrophages were isolated from 8 – 12 week old female BALB/c mice. Three ml of thioglycollate medium was injected intraperitoneally causing peritonitis in the following days. Four to five days past injection, mice were euthanized by isoflurane inhalation, sanitized with 70% ethanol and abdominal fur removed. Five ml of sterile ice cold PBS was injected into the peritoneal cavity and subsequently aspirated, now containing inflammatory cells. The PBS injection and aspiration was repeated 2 - 3 times until aspirated solution appeared clear indicating a decreased number of cells. Then, the PBS/cell solution was centrifuged at 1200 rpm for 5 min, PBS removed, the cell pellet re-suspended in complete growth medium, and macrophages cultured at 37 °C for further use.

3 RESULTS

3.1 D-DT in Apoptosis

Apoptosis is crucial for host survival and has been suggested to limit inflammatory responses (69). Prevention of cell death by MIF is well documented and a number of studies have been published to date on MIF's molecular mechanisms in various models of apoptosis. MIF has been shown to protect cells from apoptosis by preventing cytoplasmic p53 accumulation (62, 69) and by stimulating anti-apoptotic proteins (70). Thus, it was one goal of this thesis to investigate D-DT's effects on apoptosis. Therefore, human D-DT and murine D-DT cDNAs were first cloned into mammalian expression vectors. Subsequently, fibroblasts and macrophages were transfected with these generated plasmids. Protein overexpression was confirmed by Western blotting and the effect of D-DT was measured after apoptosis induction in an *in vitro* model.

3.1.1 Cloning of D-DT into Mammalian Expression Vectors

The first step was to generate human and murine D-DT plasmid constructs for specific D-DT protein overexpression in mammalian cells. Hence, hD-DT and mD-DT cDNAs were directly inserted into the plasmid vector pcDNA™3.1/V5-His-TOPO® using the method of TA Cloning. For PCR, primers were designed with a 3' stop codon, so that hD-DT and mD-DT were expressed as native proteins. For TA Cloning, *Taq* polymerase was used which has a nontemplate-dependent terminal transferase activity that adds a single deoxyadenosine (A) to the 3' end of PCR products. The linearized vector possesses single, overhanging 3' deoxythymidine (T) residues and, therefore, allows PCR inserts to ligate efficiently with the vector. Moreover, topoisomerase is covalently bound to the vector, helping to efficiently clone PCR products.

Transformants were analyzed for the correct orientation of the PCR product by DNA sequencing, and then transfected into mammalian cells for expression.

3.1.2 D-DT is Overexpressed in Cos-7 Fibroblasts

3.1.2.1 GFP Transfection Rate of 70%

Mammalian Cos-7 fibroblasts were transfected with MIF, D-DT or GFP plasmid. GFP served as a reporter gene indicating success of transfection, because the resulting protein exhibits bright green fluorescence when exposed to blue light at a wavelength of 395 nm under a fluorescent microscope. The fibroblast transfection rate was estimated to be approximately 70% (Figure 10).

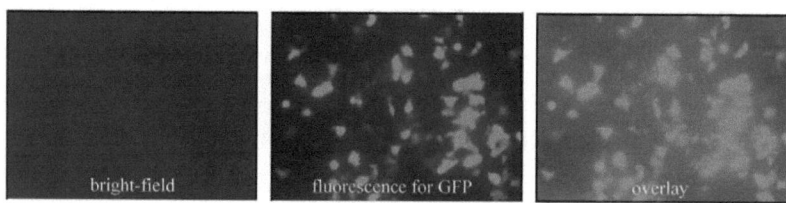

Figure 10: GFP detection in Cos-7 fibroblasts. Cos-7 fibroblasts were transfected with GFP plasmid using Lipofectamine 2000. Prior to transfection, GFP plasmid (final concentration: 0.016 g/l) and Lipofectamine 2000 (final concentration: 0.04 g/l) were diluted in Opti-MEM 1 Reduced Serum medium and incubated at room temperature for 5 min. Dilutions were combined in a 1:1 ratio and further incubated for 20 min. Then, 100 µl of DNA/Lipofectamine 2000 complexes were added to 90% confluent Cos-7 cells, which were cultured on a 24-well plate in complete growth medium without antibiotics. Subsequently, cells were incubated at 37 °C and imaged 48 h later. Green fluorescence indicates GFP-expressing fibroblasts due to successful plasmid transfection. The transfection rate was estimated to be approximately 70%. *Left panel*: bright-field. *Middle panel*: fluorescence for GFP. *Right panel*: overlay. A representative experiment is shown.

3.1.2.2 3.8-fold Overexpression of D-DT in Fibroblasts

Next, I confirmed D-DT protein overexpression in Cos-7 fibroblasts. Cells were transfected with MIF or D-DT plasmids as described for GFP transfection in Figure 10. Twenty-four h and 48 h after transfection, cells were lysed and proteins detected by Western blotting.

D-DT plasmid transfection of Cos-7 fibroblasts resulted in 3.7-fold overexpression of D-DT protein levels 24 h later (Figure 11). Forty-eight h post transfection, cytosolic D-DT protein content was detected to be 3.8-fold higher than control. These results are consistent with MIF protein levels as a 5.1-fold and a 4.1-fold increase of MIF content was observed in MIF plasmid transfected cells 24 h and 48 h after transfection.

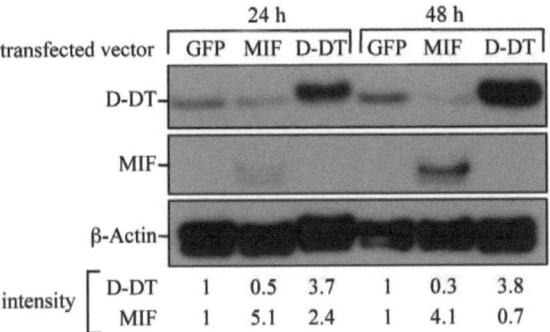

Figure 11: Overexpression of D-DT and MIF in Cos-7 fibroblasts. Cos-7 fibroblasts were transfected with MIF, D-DT plasmid or a control plasmid (GFP). Cells were lysed and total cell protein extracts were subjected to Western blot analysis detecting MIF and D-DT 24 h and 48 h after transfection. Below each Western blot, the respective band densitometry analysis performed with ImageJ software is shown. The amount of specific signal for MIF and D-DT was corrected for sample loading. The value for the 'GFP' condition 24 h and 48 h after transfection was set as 1.

3.1.3 D-DT is Overexpressed in RAW 264.7 Macrophages

3.1.3.1 GFP Transfection Rate of 35%

Nucleofection, which is based on the physical method of electroporation, was used to transfer MIF, D-DT or GFP plasmid into RAW 264.7 macrophages. Fluorescence microscopy of transfected cells allowed the monitoring of DNA transfer efficiency. A transfection rate of 35% was estimated by cell counting (Figure 12).

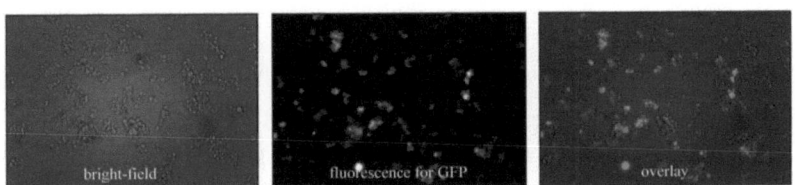

Figure 12: GFP detection in RAW 264.7 macrophages. Cells were nucleofected with GFP plasmid and 48 h later analyzed by fluorescence microscopy. Transfection efficiency was estimated to be 35%. Before transfection, RAW 264.7 macrophages were cultured in complete growth medium. Following dislodgement from the flask, cell pellets of aliquots of 2×10^6 cells were generated by centrifugation. Cell pellets were resuspended in 100 µl Nucleofector Solution V, combined with 2 µg GFP plasmid and transferred to an Amaxa certified cuvette. Nucleofector program D-032 was selected for

transfection. Immediately following nucleofection, macrophages were transferred into 6-well plates containing pre-warmed culture medium at a final concentration of 1x10⁶ cells/ml. Subsequently, cells were incubated at 37 °C. *Left panel*: bright-field. *Middle panel*: fluorescence for GFP. *Right panel*: overlay. A representative experiment is shown.

3.1.3.2   1.4-fold Overexpression of D-DT in Macrophages

Transient transfection of RAW 264.7 macrophages was generated by electroporation and overexpression analyzed by Western blotting 48 h post transfection. No increase of MIF protein levels was observed in MIF-transfected cells (Figure 13A). However, D-DT protein was measured to be 1.4-fold overexpressed in D-DT-transfected cells compared to control cells (Figure 13B). Of note, endogenous MIF and D-DT are visualized in GFP-transfected cells.

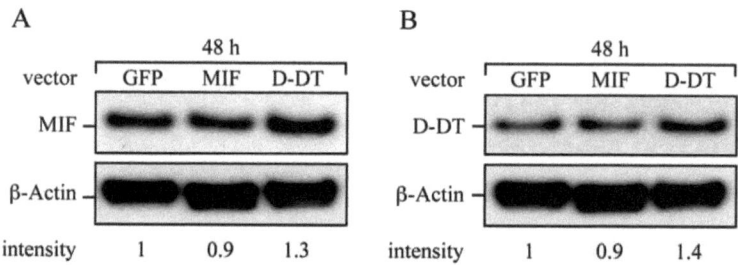

Figure 13: Analysis of MIF and D-DT content in RAW 264.7 macrophages. Cells were transfected with MIF, D-DT plasmid or control plasmid (GFP) and analyzed for MIF (**A**) and D-DT (**B**) overexpression by Western blotting 48 h after transfection. The bands visualized via Western blot were subjected to band densitometry analysis with ImageJ software. The amount of specific signal for MIF and D-DT was corrected for sample loading. The value for the 'GFP' condition was set as 1.

3.1.4 D-DT Does Not Protect from Apoptosis

After successfully generating a D-DT plasmid and confirming plasmid transfection and protein overexpression, my next objective was to determine, whether D-DT influences apoptosis. Following plasmid transfection, protein levels increased in macrophages accordingly and successive apoptosis studies were performed. Methodically, transfected RAW 264.7 macrophages were stimulated with the NO donor SNP and the rate of apoptosis measured by the detection of nucleosomes. As shown in Figure 14, overexpression of D-DT in macrophages did not reduce the level of apoptosis. Conversely, overexpression of MIF in likewise stimulated macrophages led to a decrease of apoptosis rate similar to that of GFP-transfected non-stimulated cells. This is in agreement with prior reports, which demonstrated that MIF protects macrophages from NO-induced apoptosis by preventing p53 accumulation (62, 69) and through PI3K/Akt signaling pathway (70, 72). However, these results suggest that D-DT does not protect transfected macrophages from SNP-induced apoptosis. Therefore, these reports provide first evidence of opposing actions of D-DT and MIF, and might distinguish D-DT's effects from those of MIF.

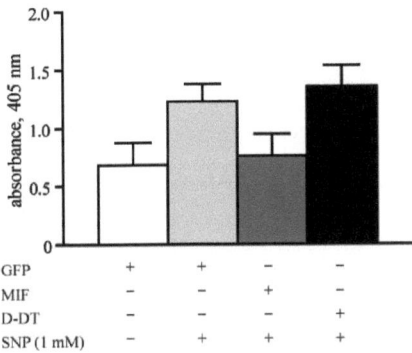

Figure 14: D-DT has no anti-apoptotic function. RAW 264.7 macrophages were transfected with D-DT plasmid or control plasmids (GFP or MIF). 48 h post transfection, apoptosis was induced by 1 mM SNP and cells incubated for 4 h. Apoptotic levels were measured by detecting the formation of nucleosomes. Results are expressed as mean±S.E. of three independent experiments. No statistical significance could be determined, p>0.05.

3.2 D-DT Enhances Cell Viability

Apart from its anti-apoptotic functions, MIF has also been implicated in maintenance of cell viability and survival and, thus, in the prolongation of inflammatory reactions in response to invading pathogens. *In vivo* LPS administration leads to greater production of pro-inflammatory cytokines (TNFα, IL-1β, and PGE$_2$) in wildtype mice compared to MIF-deficient mice (69). Of note, MIF was also shown to mostly act pro-proliferative (*e.g.*, by promoting integrin-dependent cell cycle progression) (145). Additionally, human tumors (*e.g.*, colorectal or prostatic adenocarcinoma cells) had increased MIF levels, suggesting MIF's pro-tumorigenic activity (31, 32). As with MIF, it seemed important to gain a broader understanding of the role D-DT plays in cell viability and, thus, to determine whether D-DT affects cell death or leads to cell survival. Herein, D-DT's effect on macrophage viability was addressed.

In an *in vitro* assay, stimulation of peritoneal macrophages with recombinant D-DT resulted in a higher level of cell viability compared to control (Figure 15). This increase was more pronounced than MIF-induced progression of macrophage viability, indicating quantitative differences between the effects of MIF and D-DT. Interestingly, adding MIF and D-DT simultaneously to macrophages led to an even higher increase of cell viability. These data point to a potential viability-supporting function of D-DT that is even more distinct than that of MIF, and also suggest additive effects of MIF and D-DT.

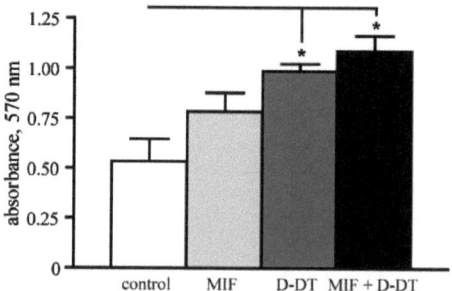

Figure 15: D-DT enhances macrophage viability. Peritoneal macrophages were collected from 8-12 weeks old BALB/c mice 4-5 days after thioglycollate-induced peritonitis. 24 h past isolation, macrophages (1×10^6/ml) were stimulated with the indicated recombinant proteins for 2 h (final concentration: 50 ng/ml) and cell viability assessed by photometrical measurement of tetrazolium salt reduction. Results are expressed as mean±S.E. of three independent experiments. Statistical significance was determined for D-DT and MIF + D-DT treated cells against untreated cells by Student's t-test, *p<0.05.

3.3 Tautomerization of *p*-Hydroxyphenylpyruvate

MIF catalyzes the tautomerization of the non-physiological substrate HPP (137). Its overall three-dimensional structure, especially the protein's amino terminal region around Pro1, is crucial for this enzymatic activity (122). This catalytic base is conserved in D-DT, resulting in similar tautomerase activity. Because D-DT has been identified as a structural homologue of MIF, and thus as a member of the MIF/tautomerase superfamily (135), it was of special interest to investigate D-DT's catalytic activity on HPP continuatively in close comparison to MIF. Moreover, the active site of MIF around Pro1 has been associated with its pro-inflammatory actions (123-125). Therefore, prototypic small molecule inhibitors have been designed that bind to the protein's amino terminal region and, thus, block MIF's effects. Co-effects or interference of these inhibitors with D-DT, specifically with D-DT's tautomerase activity or D-DT's potential downstream actions, have not been reported to date.

Taken together, these previous findings suggested that it would be beneficial to further investigate MIF's and D-DT's tautomerase activity in a comparative manner. This thesis focused specifically on quantitatively comparing D-DT's and MIF's enzymatic activity on the one hand, and the effects on D-DT of two of MIF's small molecular inhibitors, 4-IPP and ISO-1, on the other. Assessing the rate of enzymatic tautomerization of the substrate HPP in the presence of different inhibitor concentrations served this purpose. Substrate turnover was measured photometrically over the course of 3 min.

3.3.1 Human and Murine D-DT Tautomerase HPP

A direct comparison of human MIF's, human D-DT's and murine D-DT's tautomerase activity was performed using the HPP tautomerase assay (Figure 16A). Comparing their ability to catalyze the tautomerization of HPP revealed that human MIF has the highest enzymatic activity (hMIF = 4.3 ± 1.1 $\Delta305nm/min/\mu M$). Human D-DT possessed only 11% of human MIF's enzymatic ability, whereas murine D-DT achieved 76% of the tautomerase activity of human MIF (hD-DT = 0.5 ± 0.1 $\Delta305nm/min/\mu M$, and mD-DT = 3.3 ± 1.5 $\Delta305nm/min/\mu M$). These results confirmed the tautomerase activity of all three proteins and substantiated the HPP tautomerase assay as an adjuvant tool for further inhibitory studies of this enzymatic activity.

3.3.2 D-DT is Partially Sensitive to MIF Tautomerase Inhibitors

My next objective was to use the same HPP tautomerase assay to investigate whether human D-DT and murine D-DT are sensitive to human MIF-catalytic site inhibitors. I studied the inhibitory effects of 4-IPP and ISO-1, two of the many small molecular antagonists of MIF's enzymatic active site reported, on the biological activities of human MIF, human D-DT and murine D-DT. 4-IPP served as a suicide substrate for

MIF, resulting in the covalent modification of the catalytically active N-terminal proline (127). The competitive inhibitor ISO-1 was one of the first discovered MIF antagonists and is the best characterized. It reversibly binds to MIF and also interferes with MIF's biological functions *in vitro* and *in vivo* (81, 123).

Combining human MIF and 4-IPP at a 1:1 ratio led to a pronounced decrease of human MIF's enzymatic activity (95%) (Figure 16B). At higher inhibitor concentrations (1:1 and 1:5 ratios), 4-IPP abolished human MIF's enzymatic activity. Likewise, 4-IPP significantly inhibited the tautomerase activity of both human D-DT and murine D-DT, but with a greater inhibitory effect on murine D-DT. A 1:1 murine D-DT/4-IPP ratio was sufficient to reduce the enzymatic activity significantly, whereas a 10-fold 4-IPP excess was needed for the same reduction of human D-DT. Next, the competitive inhibitor ISO-1 inhibited human MIF significantly when added in 100-, 1000- or 10,000-fold molar excess (Figure 16C). In contrast, human D-DT's and murine D-DT's activity was not affected. In summary, these findings suggested that both human D-DT and murine D-DT are susceptible to the inhibitory effects of 4-IPP, however, at a reduced rate. ISO-1 obtains a selective interaction with the human MIF tautomerase site.

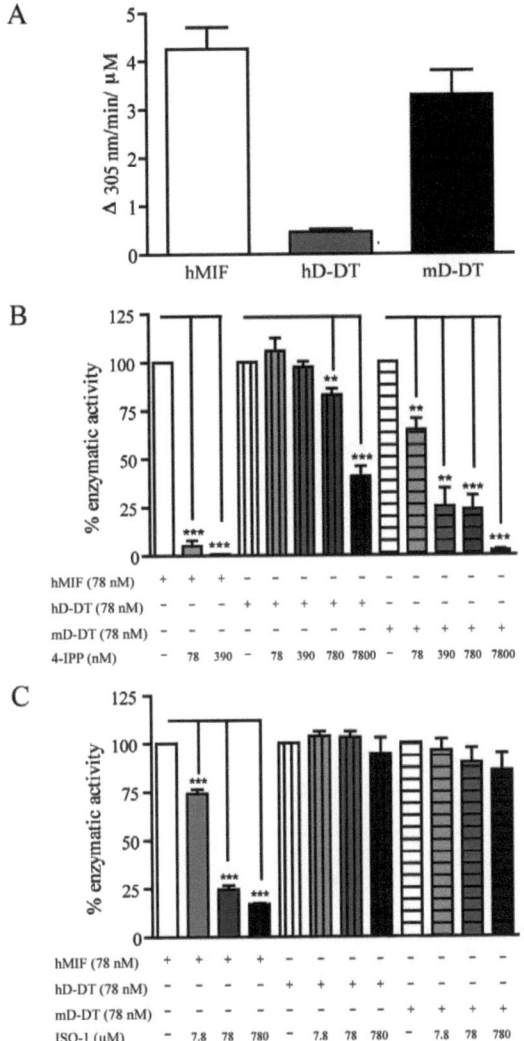

Figure 16: Tautomerization activity of human MIF, human D-DT, and murine D-DT measured with the substrate HPP. A) The enzymatic activity of the protein (78 nM) was measured by the difference in absorption at 305 nm over the course of 3 min. Data are mean±SD of six independent experiments. **B)** The small molecule inhibitor 4-IPP was pre-incubated for 10 min at room temperature with human MIF, human D-DT or murine D-DT at increasing concentrations. Data are mean±SD of triplicate independent measurements. **C)** The small molecule inhibitor ISO-1 was pre-incubated for 10 min at room temperature with human MIF, human D-DT or murine D-DT at 100-, 1000- or 10,000-fold molar excess, respectively. Data are mean±SD of triplicate independent measurements. The p values were calculated by Student's t-test (protein vs. protein + inhibitor), ***$p<0.001$, **$p<0.01$.

3.4 Neutralization of D-DT Protects Mice from LPS-Shock

The LPS-shock model has frequently been used to investigate MIF's effects in acute, severe inflammatory responses as measured by mice survival and mortality. Following LPS challenge, MIF is rapidly released from immune cells and increased MIF-levels are observed in the blood circulation (11, 13, 30). Similarly, it has been reported that bone marrow-derived macrophages secrete D-DT in response to LPS (116). The pattern of release of D-DT is similar to that reported of MIF, exhibiting a bell-shaped curve peaking at 16 h after pro-inflammatory stimulus. Therefore, in this thesis, it was of interest to validate whether neutralization of D-DT, like neutralization of MIF, protects mice from LPS shock. The herein administered specific polyclonal antibody had previously been reported not to show any cross-reactivity to MIF (116). Figure 17 illustrates that, indeed, administration of anti-D-DT antibody significantly increased survival rate from 20% to 79% following challenge of an LD_{80} dose of LPS. This degree of protection is comparable to what was achieved previously with anti-MIF (11).

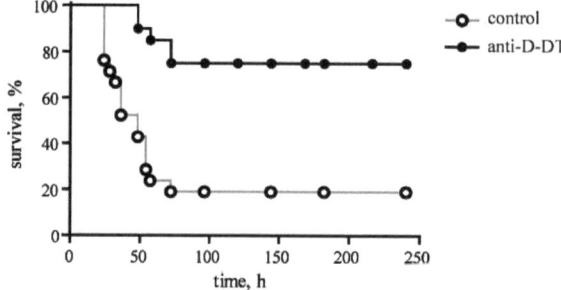

Figure 17: Neutralization of D-DT protects mice in a model of lethal endotoxemia. Female BALB/c mice (6-8 weeks) were intraperitoneally injected with 200 µl of anti-mD-DT serum or control serum. Two h later, LPS was injected (20 mg/kg). Mice were observed for 2 weeks. Data points are from three independent experiments, each of which included 5-10 mice per treatment group. Survival was 75% (15 of 20) in mice treated with anti-D-DT antibody, and 19% (4 of 21) in mice treated with control antibody. P<0.0001, Kaplan-Meier.

4 DISCUSSION

In 1993, a new enzyme that specifically tautomerizes the *D*-isomer of dopachrome was found in human tissue (132). It was named D-DT due to this first discovery. Two years later, cloning and sequencing of a cDNA encoding D-DT disclosed sequence homology with MIF (146). Sugimoto *et al.* determined the X-ray crystal structure of D-DT with a result of strong structural homology between MIF and D-DT (135). As a consequence, it was presumed that D-DT might play a similar physiological role to the immunoregulator MIF. A few observations support the hypothesis that MIF and D-DT share some biological abilities. First, the mRNA and protein levels of D-DT are unchanged in *mif* knockout cells compared to wildtype control cells (116). Second, both proteins are released constitutively at a low level and are efficiently secreted after stimulation with LPS from macrophages. Moreover, the depletion of either MIF or D-DT by siRNA results in similar effects, precisely in the transcriptional regulation of IL-8, both involving the receptor CD74 (140).

More recently, studies of B cell apoptosis and monocyte arrest showed that neutralization or genetic deletion of MIF does not completely abrogate downstream activation responses (20, 147). The deletion of the MIF receptor CD74 produces a more pronounced phenotype than MIF deficiency. This observation may be explained by a second MIF-like ligand, which possibly may be D-DT (87). As there is very little knowledge about the physiological role of D-DT to date, further studies would be useful to elucidate D-DT's precise role.

4.1 D-DT was Overexpressed for Apoptosis Studies

4.1.1 TA Cloning Generates D-DT Plasmid

Prior to functional studies of D-DT (*e.g.*, its effect on apoptosis) the D-DT cDNA was cloned into a mammalian expression vector. Mammalian cells were subsequently transfected with the newly generated plasmids and protein overexpression confirmed. In this thesis, TA Cloning was used to generate D-DT plasmid constructs. It is an easy and quick subcloning technique that clones PCR amplified inserts directly into linearized vectors without the use of restriction enzymes (148). The complementary base pairs thymine (T; at both ends of the linearized vector) and adenine (A; at both ends of the PCR product) hybridize and become ligated together. Because no restriction sites are needed, shorter primers can be utilized, which facilitates the procedure. On the downside, no directional cloning is guaranteed and the gene is inserted in reverse direction in 50% of all successfully cloned vectors. Consequently, DNA sequencing is needed to confirm correct orientation of the gene.

4.1.2 Lipofectamine 2000 Transfects Fibroblasts

In this thesis, the reagent Lipofectamine 2000 was applied for Cos-7 fibroblast transfection. It is a cationic liposome formulation that functions by forming a complex with net negatively charged nucleic acid, allowing it to overcome the electrostatic repulsion of the cell membrane and, thus, to be taken up by the cell (149). With the help of Lipofectamine 2000, plasmid DNA reaches the nucleus of the cell, becomes accessible to the transcriptional machinery and, thus, D-DT is expressed. Also, in actively dividing cells, such as Cos-7 fibroblasts, transfected DNA simply becomes trapped in the nucleus following the reassembly of the nuclear envelope at the end of mitosis. However, Lipofectamine 2000 has been shown to promote penetration of DNA through intact nuclear envelopes. It provides a rather chemical than physical method of cell transfection and, thus, is considered to be gentler, which results in high transfection efficiencies and high levels of transgene expression without excessive cytotoxicity. In Cos-7 fibroblasts, a transfection rate of approximately 70% was achieved, which was indicated by GFP fluorescence. However, a few scientists recently supposed that GFP fluorescence overestimates transfection efficiency. Subsequent Western blotting confirmed protein overexpression by visualizing 3.7-fold and 3.8-fold increased D-DT and 5.1-fold and 4.1-fold increased MIF levels, 24 h and 48 h after fibroblast transfection. These results emphasize Lipofectamine 2000's utility in fibroblast transfection, as a high transfection rate of viable cells results in high protein overexpression.

4.1.3 Macrophage Transfection Results from Nucleofection

In contrast to Cos-7 fibroblasts, RAW 264.7 macrophages were transiently transfected with plasmids using the Nucleofector technology, which transfers plasmid DNA directly into the cell nucleus. It uses a combination of an electric pulse and the appropriate, cell-type specific media, which together decrease the toxicity of the otherwise harsh method of electroporation leading to excessive cell death (150). Nucleofection promotes efficient transfection of difficult-to-transfect cells, such as immune cells, when gentler methods give poor results. Nevertheless, cell death is more frequent during nucleofection than during lipid-based methods. In this thesis, macrophages were transfected by nucleofection and a transfection rate of 35% was estimated by cell counting. Subsequent protein detection by Western blotting could not confirm increased MIF levels. Nevertheless, it demonstrated a slight overexpression of D-DT (1.4-fold increased D-DT levels), which was lower compared to fibroblast transfection by Lipofectamine 2000, as cell mortality rate was higher and transfection efficiency significantly lower in nucleofection-transfected cells.

4.2 MIF Acts Anti-Apoptotically

Previous studies have linked MIF's pro-inflammatory actions to its ability to protect immune cells from apoptosis and, thus, to prolong the inflammatory response. So far, several mechanisms of MIF action have been described: MIF prevents p53 accumulation in the cytoplasm (62, 69) and cytochrome c release from mitochondria (71). It also promotes the anti-apoptotic factors Bcl-2 (70) and NF-κB (72). In order to study D-DT's functional properties in comparison to MIF, it was indispensable to establish a reliable experimental setup that was consistent with previously reported signaling ways of MIF. Such a system would allow confirmation or refutation of D-DT's functional similarities to MIF, which are suggested by structural homology and previous reports of action of both proteins.

To this end, macrophages were first transfected with either MIF or D-DT plasmids using nucleofection. As discussed before, cell transfection led to cell death and stress of the surviving macrophages, that ingested the plasmid. Hence, a transfection rate of 35% and a 1.4-fold overexpression of D-DT were achieved. This is consistent with previously reported results of experiments using identical materials and experimental conditions. Following transfection, apoptosis was induced by the NO donor sodium nitroprusside. Since Hudson *et al.* and Mitchell *et al.* reported that MIF protects macrophages from NO-induced apoptosis by preventing p53 accumulation (62, 69) it was assumed that MIF decreases apoptotic levels in this analogous experimental setup. Subsequently, the level of macrophage apoptosis was measured by detecting the formation of nucleosomes in the cytoplasm. As expected, incubation of control-transfected macrophages with SNP led to increased apoptotic levels compared to non-SNP treated cells. Second, MIF-transfected macrophages showed almost baseline apoptotic levels. However, previous Western blotting did not show MIF to be overexpressed following plasmid transfection. The fact that apoptotic levels are higher in SNP-treated control-transfected cells than in MIF-transfected macrophages indicates that the physiological MIF content alone is not sufficient to reduce apoptosis to baseline. Various reasons might account for the unsuccessful detection of overexpressed MIF levels. One of them might be that the blotting membrane was not able to detect overexpressed MIF levels due to limits of its sensitivity or to its saturation. Of note, physical cell stress by nucleofection did not diminish MIF's effect on apoptosis, as indicated by lower rate of apoptosis. These results are consistent with previous reports about MIF's functions.

4.2.1 D-DT does not Diminish Apoptosis

In contrast to MIF, D-DT did not decrease the level of NO-induced apoptosis in macrophages, even despite 1.4-fold protein overexpression. Apoptotic levels of D-DT transfected macrophages were comparable to those of control-transfected cells, which had been treated with SNP. It might be speculated that higher concentrations of D-DT are needed to protect from apoptosis, that D-DT does not impact NO-mediated apoptosis induction (or even apoptosis) at all, or that the nucleofection treatment of macrophages might have altered cell function in a way that made them less susceptible to subsequent D-DT effects. Whatever the reason, apoptotic levels of D-DT transfected macrophages remained high.

This is the first report on D-DT's effect on apoptosis. To validate these results, it would be useful to investigate D-DT's role in various experimental setups. The effects of D-DT can be investigated in knockdown experiments with *e.g.*, siRNA, or by using different cell lines, different ways of apoptosis induction, or by the administration of small molecule inhibitors. Also, its effects on different pro- and anti-apoptotic proteins, such as *e.g.*, p53, Bcl-2 or NF-κB, can be determined, which would possibly elucidate D-DT's molecular mechanisms of action. Furthermore, detecting the influence of recombinant D-DT (instead of overexpressed D-DT) on the level of apoptosis may provide a beneficial tool to investigate D-DT's abilities. Nevertheless, my data provide first insights into the biological functions of D-DT.

4.3 D-DT Enhances Macrophage Viability

Previous studies have demonstrated that MIF prolongs inflammatory responses by enhancing viability and survival of immune cells (69). MIF causes macrophages to release higher levels of pro-inflammatory cytokines, such as TNFα, IL-1β, and PGE$_2$. MIF is also involved in cell cycle progression through sustained ERK activation and cyclin D1 expression (145). However, MIF also interacts with JAB1 (75). Quantitative analysis of MIF level showed that it is overexpressed in human tumors, indicating tumor-supportive and, thus, pro-proliferative functions of MIF (31, 32). So far, little is known about D-DT's role in cell viability, the prolongation of inflammatory responses, or cell cycle regulation. So far, only a few publications have linked D-DT to proliferation. Coleman *et al.* suggested a biological role for MIF and D-DT in NSCLC by reporting that both proteins were required for expression of proangiogenic factors, such as CXCL8 and VEGF (140). Moreover, D-DT has been reported to affect colorectal cancer disease progression through COX-2 expression (141). Aside from those, no specific studies of D-DT's effect on cell viability, or sustained inflammation have been reported to date.

To fill this void, peritoneal macrophage viability was assessed *in vitro* in response to MIF, D-DT, or simultaneous stimulation by recombinant proteins. It was observed that MIF-treatment resulted in increased cell viability, which is in accord with previous reports on MIF's functions. Interestingly, stimulation of macrophages with recombinant D-DT led to a more pronounced viability compared to that of MIF. This observation indicates that D-DT, like MIF, may enhance cell viability and survival. It further proposes that D-DT's effects may be more distinct compared to those of MIF. Therefore, it might be suspected that D-DT favors prolonged inflammatory responses similar to MIF. However, as these are one of the first reports on D-DT's functions, further studies are needed to validate this statement. It would be interesting to study whether D-DT also leads to the release of pro-inflammatory cytokines, resulting in enhanced inflammatory responses. In this case, D-DT's effects on macrophages as well as on other immune cells should be investigated, as this would give more precise insight into D-DT's regulatory role in inflammation. Moreover, it remains uncertain which signal transduction pathways might explain this result, as there is very little knowledge about D-DT's intracellular effects at all. For example, D-DT might enhance macrophage viability due to its downstream effect on ERK or p53. Another possibility is that D-DT influences completely different cellular factors or mechanisms that have not yet been discovered. A study of D-DT's intracellular mechanisms shows that D-DT-induced CXCL8 expression requires JNK, c-JUN and AP-1 as well as the CD74 receptor (140). The discovery that CD74 is important for D-DT's downstream effects raises the question whether D-DT, like MIF, is a CD74 ligand. Recent observations strengthen the hypothesis that CD74 might have a second ligand, because deletion of the receptor abrogates downstream MIF effects more significantly than neutralization or genetic deletion of MIF alone (147, 151). In 2011, it was demonstrated that D-DT binds CD74 with high affinity, as well as the intracellular transcription regulator JAB1 (87). However, it remains for further investigation whether binding of D-DT to CD74 is involved in signaling leading to enhanced cell viability.

Moreover, my data show that incubation of macrophages with MIF and D-DT simultaneously increased cell viability even more compared to treatment with only one protein. These findings may suggest additive effects of MIF and D-DT and, thus, might lead to the conclusion that both proteins support each other in enhancing cell viability. However, subsequent experiments are needed as well to confirm this possibility.

Although all of these conclusions support the possibility of D-DT having a viability-supporting function, the experimental methods need to be considered. The MTT proliferation assay measures cell viability by colorimetric detection of tetrazole salt metabolism in mitochondria. As a result, altered mitochondrial function, potentially caused by D-DT, might mimic cell viability and might lead to overestimated viability levels. Further studies of D-DT in different experimental settings are necessary in order to further evaluate its functions.

4.4 MIF and D-DT are Structural Homologues

4.4.1 Quantitative Differences in Tautomerase Activity

MIF and D-DT have been shown to share a similar three-dimensional structure and were, thus, classified as members of the MIF/tautomerase superfamily (115). Due to their structural homology, both proteins were identified as enzymes catalyzing the tautomerization of *D*-dopachrome and HPP (136, 137). However, no detailed quantitative studies and comparisons of MIF's and D-DT's enzymatic activities have been performed to date. In this thesis, I report that human D-DT's enzymatic activity on HPP is approximately 10 times lower than that measured for MIF, whereas the tautomerase activity of the murine D-DT is approximately 25% less than that of MIF. These findings suggest that differences, most likely the slight structural differences, exist between these three proteins and cause enzymatic distinction.

It previously was shown that the N-terminal proline which resides within a hydrophobic, substrate-binding pocket (122, 152, 153) functions as a catalytic base in the tautomerization of *D*-dopachrome and HPP (121). The proline residue is well conserved between MIF and D-DT, although a detailed comparison revealed significant differences in the environment around the active site, the intersubunit contacts, and the charge distribution on the molecular surface (135). In human MIF the active site pockets are positively charged, although non-charged regions also have been reported. In contrast, human D-DT shows a widely distributed negatively charged surface. Only the regions around the active sites are positively charged. In human MIF five distinct amino acids are implicated in HPP substrate contact: Pro1, Lys32, Ile64, Tyr95 and Asn97 (122). Human D-DT shares three of these five amino acids (Pro1, Lys32 and Ile64) with human MIF. However, two residues are absent. Tyr95 is replaced by Ile95, and Asn97 by Ile97. Moreover, MIF and D-DT show differences in the theoretical isoelectric points of their protein sequences. Human MIF possesses an isoelectric point of pH 7.7, whereas human D-DT and murine D-DT carry no net electric charge in a slightly acidic environment (human D-DT: pH 6.7 versus murine D-DT: pH 6.1). At pH 6.2 during the HPP tautomerase assay, MIF's and D-DT's amino acid residues show a specific charge, which results in either facilitating or aggravating substrate turnover. Taken together, these slight structural differences might suggest possible explanations for the diverse interaction of the substrate HPP with the catalytic sites of the proteins and, thus, the different enzymatic activities of human MIF, human D-DT and murine D-DT.

4.4.2 Tautomerase Inhibitors Affect D-DT to Lesser Extent

In addition, the prior reported slight structural differences between MIF and D-DT might as well account for the diverse inhibition of their tautomerase activity by 4-IPP and ISO-1. These two proteins have been characterized as catalytic inhibitors of MIF, which operate by blocking its amino-terminal tautomerase region (123, 127). As previously described in this thesis, the covalent MIF inhibitor 4-IPP reduces D-DT's tautomerase activity significantly (albeit at higher inhibitor concentrations compared to MIF), whereas the competitive MIF inhibitor ISO-1 is selective for MIF. These results indicate that low 4-IPP concentrations result in augmented inhibition of MIF, while excessive use of 4-IPP inhibits both proteins. The different inhibitory properties of ISO-1 on MIF and D-DT might provide the possibility of specific inhibition of MIF's enzymatic activity while leaving D-DT unaffected. This could provide a useful tool for isolating and investigating D-DT's effects in future research challenges. This also suggests the possibility of developing therapeutically beneficial pharmacological inhibitors in situations where specific inhibition of one protein, but not the other, is intended.

4.4.3 Enzymatic Inhibitors Might Impact Biological Function

The tautomerization site centered around Pro1 in MIF has been linked to some of its pro-inflammatory actions, such as the counter-regulation of glucocorticoids (123), neutrophil priming (124) and the upregulation of metalloproteinases-1 and -3 (123-125). Although this motif is conserved in D-DT, differences in the tautomerase activity associated with this region are apparent. The lower tautomerase activity of D-DT might suggest qualitative or quantitative differences in the biological function of MIF and D-DT.

ISO-1 has been shown to inhibit some of MIF's pro-inflammatory actions, such as the production of TNFα, PGE$_2$ and COX-2 *in vitro* (123), and protection against death in an *in vivo* mouse model of endotoxic shock (81). Therefore, it might be suggested that ISO-1 does not have these effects on D-DT. As, to date, D-DT's biological actions are almost completely unknown these aspects remain to be subject for further validation in future.

4.5 Neutralization of D-DT Protects Mice from Endotoxic Shock

Various studies have identified MIF in host response to LPS, the main virulence factor of Gram-negative bacteria. In a murine model of LPS-induced endotoxemia, MIF is rapidly released into the bloodstream, presenting a bell-shaped increase of MIF concentration that peaks at 8 - 20 hours after LPS challenge (11, 13, 30). Utilizing the same endotoxic shock model, injection of recombinant MIF increased mice mortality, whereas its neutralization led to mice survival. These results are in accord with reports of pro-inflammatory actions of MIF and further demonstrate its immunoregulatory role. Recently, D-DT has been identified as a protein released from immune cells in response to LPS (116). Likewise, D-DT's release pattern is similar to that of MIF, peaking at 16 hours post pro-inflammatory stimulus. However, cultured macrophages release 20-fold more MIF than D-DT. These observations describe similarities in the release of MIF and D-DT in response to LPS. However, no data on D-DT's role in an *in vivo* endotoxic shock model has been published to date.

In this work, I show that an anti-D-DT antibody protects mice from LPS shock, which is analogous to previous reports of MIF neutralization. A specific polyclonal antibody targeting murine D-DT was used that has been reported not to have any cross reactivity to MIF (116). Hence, these results suggest that D-DT might play a similar pro-inflammatory function as MIF. However, these are the first reports of neutralization of D-DT and subsequent studies should be conducted to further substantiate these results. For example, it would be useful to investigate whether neutralization of D-DT leads to reduced pro-inflammatory cytokine production as has been reported for MIF. Neutralization of MIF by ISO-1 or absence of MIF in $mif^{-/-}$ mice inhibited TNFα release from macrophages after LPS administration (18, 81). Very recently, Merk *et al.* reported that D-DT neutralization prior to LPS injection led to a significant reduction of the circulating concentrations of pro-inflammatory cytokines (TNFα, IL-1β, INFγ, IL-12p70), as well as to an increased concentration of anti-inflammatory IL-10 (87).

Moreover, mice survival in experiments using other means of D-DT neutralization (*e.g.*, the deletion of the *D-dt* gene or the use of small molecular inhibitors) could be addressed, as various means of MIF neutralization have been shown to have positive effects on mice survival. Currently, a *D*-dt knock-out mouse is developed which will serve useful for further investigations of D-DT's functions *in vivo* (87). Regarding inhibitors, it should be noted, that ISO-1 has not been shown to inhibit D-DT's enzymatic activity. The results of this thesis suggest that pretreatment of mice with ISO-1 prior to LPS challenge will not affect D-DT-provoked mortality. However, were specific small molecular D-DT inhibitors to become available in the future, they might have the potential to increase mice survival in endotoxemia. Simultaneous specific inhibition of MIF and D-DT might have the potential to further increase mice survival. This combined neutralization of both proteins might have an additive or synergistic effect. Taken even further, these results may also have therapeutic implications in human sepsis. To gain further understanding of D-DT actions, mice mortality could additionally be observed after concurrent intraperitoneal injection of recombinant D-DT and LPS. Here, a pronounced mice mortality rate would affirm D-DT's pro-inflammatory action.

D-DT's molecular modes of action were not investigated in this thesis. However, on a molecular level MIF has been shown to upregulate TLR4 expression and, thus, to facilitate the detection of LPS and rapidly induce the production of pro-inflammatory cytokines that are essential for host defense (37, 56). Investigating the molecular cascade triggered by released D-DT in respond to LPS would provide further insight into D-DT's precise functions.

4.5.1 D-DT in Human Sepsis is Promising Research Subject

In order to transfer the results obtained in mice to humans, it would be useful to address human D-DT levels for investigation in future experiments. Similar to mouse models of endotoxemia, MIF serum levels have been shown to be significantly higher in patients suffering from severe sepsis and septic shock compared to healthy control groups (82). A correlation between disease severity and MIF levels has been observed (154). Similar results for D-DT would further underline its role in disease development in response to Gram-negative bacteria. Recently, function studies of D-DT revealed that D-DT serum levels correlate with disease severity in sepsis and invasive cancer (87). Anti-MIF treatments have been shown to be beneficial in many inflammatory diseases. Yet, my data suggest that these approaches might not be complete without considering D-DT's possible role in disease progression. Thus, studying D-DT's *in vivo* functions as well as the molecular mechanisms underlying these effects might allow for the improvement of established anti-MIF treatments in inflammatory disease.

5 Summary and Outlook

Macrophage migration inhibitory factor (MIF) is a pleiotropic immunoregulatory and pro-inflammatory cytokine, which plays a pivotal role in the pathogenesis of various acute and chronic inflammatory diseases such as septic shock, rheumatoid arthritis, or atherosclerosis. For example, endotoxemia studies in mice reveal that MIF administration decreases the survival rate, whereas neutralization of MIF improves the chances for a beneficial outcome. As mounting evidence suggests that chronic inflammation contributes towards a microenvironment that favors tumorigenesis, high MIF levels are measured in a variety of human tumors. Additionally, functional studies reveal MIF involvement in multiple aspects of tumor progression including control of cell proliferation, prevention of apoptosis, and promotion of angiogenesis. On a molecular level, MIF is released from inflammatory cells upon stimulation. Subsequently, MIF binds to its cell surface receptors, resulting in initiation of defined signaling cascades that control local and systemic immune responses. Unlike other cytokines, MIF also is a phenylpyruvate tautomerase that converts two non-physiologic enzymatic substrates, *D*-dopachrome and *p*-hydroxyphenylpyruvate (HPP). To date, possible relationships between the tautomerase and inflammatory or tumor-supportive activities of MIF remain unclear.

In 1993, *D*-dopachrome tautomerase (D-DT) was discovered during an investigation of melanogenesis. The tertiary structure of D-DT is remarkably similar to MIF, identifying D-DT as the only known eukaryotic MIF homologue discovered to date. D-DT shares MIF's tautomerase activity and, thus, both proteins are members of the MIF tautomerase superfamily. Despite D-DT's intriguing similarities to the very well studied MIF, there have been very few reports on the biological functions and mechanisms of action of D-DT. Recent studies illustrate the individual and cooperative actions of MIF and D-DT in non-small cell lung carcinoma and colorectal cancer, suggesting a role for D-DT in the progression of neoplasm. As the importance of MIF's contributions to many inflammatory and proliferative processes has now been generally accepted, interest in the biological actions of D-DT has increased. It is possible that functional characterization of D-DT implies subsequent therapeutic consequences and might improve or even complete established anti-MIF treatments.

This thesis aims at the functional characterization of D-DT. Prior to apoptotic studies, I report on cloning D-DT cDNA into a mammalian expression vector and transfecting mammalian fibroblasts and macrophages with the generated plasmid. Fluorescence microscopy and Western blotting confirm cell transfection and D-DT overexpression. My successive data demonstrates that D-DT does not exhibit anti-apoptotic effects upon nitric oxide-induced apoptosis in transfected macrophages. For the first time, this suggests contrary effects of D-DT in comparison to MIF. Yet, it is important to note that MIF acts anti-apoptotically in the same experimental setting, which is in accord with previous reports of MIF's functions. Moreover, in a subsequent cell survival study of D-DT, I was able to illustrate that D-DT enhances macrophage viability to a more pronounced extent than MIF. Interestingly, my data further show that simultaneous treatment of cells with MIF and D-DT increases macrophage viability even more, which suggests additive effects of both proteins. These observations lead to the conclusion that MIF and D-DT may not exhibit identical functions. D-DT may even have non-agonistic or antagonistic effects in certain settings. Because my results suggest additive effects of MIF and D-DT, they provide first evidence of the importance of studying MIF's and D-DT's combined actions in the future. In addition, I am able to characterize D-DT as a protein that tautomerizes the substrate HPP and, thus, possesses analog enzymatic activity to MIF. However, quantitative differences in the tautomerization rate become evident between different mammalian homologues of D-DT. Other enzymatic studies have revealed that the covalent MIF inhibitor 4-IPP also inhibits the tautomerase activity of D-DT, whereas D-DT is not susceptible to ISO-1. Taken together, these results demonstrate general enzymatic similarity between MIF and D-DT, which is most likely a consequence of previously reported structural homology. However, MIF and D-DT differ in their susceptibility to enzymatic inhibitors. Moreover, my thesis demonstrates first insight into D-DT's *in vivo* role in a murine model of endotoxic shock. I show that neutralization of D-DT has a protective effect in the LPS-shock model. This finding accords with results reported for MIF and, therefore, suggests analog functions of D-DT in this context. Taken together, my data demonstrate in most cases fairly similar, but also contrary biologic functions of MIF and D-DT. The precise therapeutic consequences of these findings were beyond the scope of this thesis, but my results provide first hints in this direction. As this is one of the first approaches to determine D-DT's role in disease, continuative investigations need to be conducted to further validate these observations.

6 References

1. Rich, A. R., Lewis, M.R. 1932. The nature of allergy in tuberculosis as revealed by tissue culture studies. *Bulletin of The Johns Hopkins Hospital* 50:115-131.
2. George, M., and J. H. Vaughan. 1962. In vitro cell migration as a model for delayed hypersensitivity. *Proc Soc Exp Biol Med* 111:514-521.
3. David, J. R. 1966. Delayed hypersensitivity in vitro: its mediation by cell-free substances formed by lymphoid cell-antigen interaction. *Proc Natl Acad Sci U S A* 56:72-77.
4. Bloom, B. R., and B. Bennett. 1966. Mechanism of a reaction in vitro associated with delayed-type hypersensitivity. *Science* 153:80-82.
5. Nathan, C. F., M. L. Karnovsky, and J. R. David. 1971. Alterations of macrophage functions by mediators from lymphocytes. *J Exp Med* 133:1356-1376.
6. Nathan, C. F., H. G. Remold, and J. R. David. 1973. Characterization of a lymphocyte factor which alters macrophage functions. *J Exp Med* 137:275-290.
7. Burmeister, G., L. Tarcsay, and C. Sorg. 1986. Generation and characterization of a monoclonal antibody (1C5) to human migration inhibitory factor (MIF). *Immunobiology* 171:461-474.
8. McInnes, A., and D. M. Rennick. 1988. Interleukin 4 induces cultured monocytes/macrophages to form giant multinucleated cells. *J Exp Med* 167:598-611.
9. Thurman, G. B., I. A. Braude, P. W. Gray, R. K. Oldham, and H. C. Stevenson. 1985. MIF-like activity of natural and recombinant human interferon-gamma and their neutralization by monoclonal antibody. *J Immunol* 134:305-309.
10. Weiser, W. Y., P. A. Temple, J. S. Witek-Giannotti, H. G. Remold, S. C. Clark, and J. R. David. 1989. Molecular cloning of a cDNA encoding a human macrophage migration inhibitory factor. *Proc Natl Acad Sci U S A* 86:7522-7526.
11. Bernhagen, J., T. Calandra, R. A. Mitchell, S. B. Martin, K. J. Tracey, W. Voelter, K. R. Manogue, A. Cerami, and R. Bucala. 1993. MIF is a pituitary-derived cytokine that potentiates lethal endotoxaemia. *Nature* 365:756-759.
12. Bernhagen, J., R. A. Mitchell, T. Calandra, W. Voelter, A. Cerami, and R. Bucala. 1994. Purification, bioactivity, and secondary structure analysis of mouse and human macrophage migration inhibitory factor (MIF). *Biochemistry* 33:14144-14155.
13. Calandra, T., J. Bernhagen, R. A. Mitchell, and R. Bucala. 1994. The macrophage is an important and previously unrecognized source of macrophage migration inhibitory factor. *J Exp Med* 179:1895-1902.
14. Calandra, T., L. A. Spiegel, C. N. Metz, and R. Bucala. 1998. Macrophage migration inhibitory factor is a critical mediator of the activation of immune cells by exotoxins of Gram-positive bacteria. *Proc Natl Acad Sci U S A* 95:11383-11388.
15. Bernhagen, J., M. Bacher, T. Calandra, C. N. Metz, S. B. Doty, T. Donnelly, and R. Bucala. 1996. An essential role for macrophage migration inhibitory

factor in the tuberculin delayed-type hypersensitivity reaction. *J Exp Med* 183:277-282.

16. Martiney, J. A., B. Sherry, C. N. Metz, M. Espinoza, A. S. Ferrer, T. Calandra, H. E. Broxmeyer, and R. Bucala. 2000. Macrophage migration inhibitory factor release by macrophages after ingestion of Plasmodium chabaudi-infected erythrocytes: possible role in the pathogenesis of malarial anemia. *Infect Immun* 68:2259-2267.

17. Calandra, T., J. Bernhagen, C. N. Metz, L. A. Spiegel, M. Bacher, T. Donnelly, A. Cerami, and R. Bucala. 1995. MIF as a glucocorticoid-induced modulator of cytokine production. *Nature* 377:68-71.

18. Bozza, M., A. R. Satoskar, G. Lin, B. Lu, A. A. Humbles, C. Gerard, and J. R. David. 1999. Targeted disruption of migration inhibitory factor gene reveals its critical role in sepsis. *J Exp Med* 189:341-346.

19. Leng, L., C. N. Metz, Y. Fang, J. Xu, S. Donnelly, J. Baugh, T. Delohery, Y. Chen, R. A. Mitchell, and R. Bucala. 2003. MIF signal transduction initiated by binding to CD74. *J Exp Med* 197:1467-1476.

20. Bernhagen, J., R. Krohn, H. Lue, J. L. Gregory, A. Zernecke, R. R. Koenen, M. Dewor, I. Georgiev, A. Schober, L. Leng, T. Kooistra, G. Fingerle-Rowson, P. Ghezzi, R. Kleemann, S. R. McColl, R. Bucala, M. J. Hickey, and C. Weber. 2007. MIF is a noncognate ligand of CXC chemokine receptors in inflammatory and atherogenic cell recruitment. *Nat Med* 13:587-596.

21. Meyer-Siegler, K. L., P. L. Vera, K. A. Iczkowski, C. Bifulco, A. Lee, P. K. Gregersen, L. Leng, and R. Bucala. 2007. Macrophage migration inhibitory factor (MIF) gene polymorphisms are associated with increased prostate cancer incidence. *Genes Immun* 8:646-652.

22. Mizue, Y., S. Ghani, L. Leng, C. McDonald, P. Kong, J. Baugh, S. J. Lane, J. Craft, J. Nishihira, S. C. Donnelly, Z. Zhu, and R. Bucala. 2005. Role for macrophage migration inhibitory factor in asthma. *Proc Natl Acad Sci U S A* 102:14410-14415.

23. Radstake, T. R., F. C. Sweep, P. Welsing, B. Franke, S. H. Vermeulen, A. Geurts-Moespot, T. Calandra, R. Donn, and P. L. van Riel. 2005. Correlation of rheumatoid arthritis severity with the genetic functional variants and circulating levels of macrophage migration inhibitory factor. *Arthritis Rheum* 52:3020-3029.

24. Baugh, J. A., S. Chitnis, S. C. Donnelly, J. Monteiro, X. Lin, B. J. Plant, F. Wolfe, P. K. Gregersen, and R. Bucala. 2002. A functional promoter polymorphism in the macrophage migration inhibitory factor (MIF) gene associated with disease severity in rheumatoid arthritis. *Genes Immun* 3:170-176.

25. Plant, B. J., C. G. Gallagher, R. Bucala, J. A. Baugh, S. Chappell, L. Morgan, C. M. O'Connor, K. Morgan, and S. C. Donnelly. 2005. Cystic fibrosis, disease severity, and a macrophage migration inhibitory factor polymorphism. *Am J Respir Crit Care Med* 172:1412-1415.

26. Bacher, M., C. N. Metz, T. Calandra, K. Mayer, J. Chesney, M. Lohoff, D. Gemsa, T. Donnelly, and R. Bucala. 1996. An essential regulatory role for macrophage migration inhibitory factor in T-cell activation. *Proc Natl Acad Sci U S A* 93:7849-7854.

27. Thiele, M., and J. Bernhagen. 2005. Link between macrophage migration inhibitory factor and cellular redox regulation. *Antioxid Redox Signal* 7:1234-1248.
28. Rossi, A. G., C. Haslett, N. Hirani, A. P. Greening, I. Rahman, C. N. Metz, R. Bucala, and S. C. Donnelly. 1998. Human circulating eosinophils secrete macrophage migration inhibitory factor (MIF). Potential role in asthma. *J Clin Invest* 101:2869-2874.
29. Takahashi, A., K. Iwabuchi, M. Suzuki, K. Ogasawara, J. Nishihira, and K. Onoe. 1999. Antisense macrophage migration inhibitory factor (MIF) prevents anti-IgM mediated growth arrest and apoptosis of a murine B cell line by regulating cell cycle progression. *Microbiol Immunol* 43:61-67.
30. Bacher, M., A. Meinhardt, H. Y. Lan, W. Mu, C. N. Metz, J. A. Chesney, T. Calandra, D. Gemsa, T. Donnelly, R. C. Atkins, and R. Bucala. 1997. Migration inhibitory factor expression in experimentally induced endotoxemia. *Am J Pathol* 150:235-246.
31. Wilson, J. M., P. L. Coletta, R. J. Cuthbert, N. Scott, K. MacLennan, G. Hawcroft, L. Leng, J. B. Lubetsky, K. K. Jin, E. Lolis, F. Medina, J. A. Brieva, R. Poulsom, A. F. Markham, R. Bucala, and M. A. Hull. 2005. Macrophage migration inhibitory factor promotes intestinal tumorigenesis. *Gastroenterology* 129:1485-1503.
32. Meyer-Siegler, K., R. A. Fattor, and P. B. Hudson. 1998. Expression of macrophage migration inhibitory factor in the human prostate. *Diagn Mol Pathol* 7:44-50.
33. Bucala, R. 2007. *MIF : most interesting factor*. World Scientific Publishing Co. Pte. Ltd., Yale University, USA.
34. Nishino, T., J. Bernhagen, H. Shiiki, T. Calandra, K. Dohi, and R. Bucala. 1995. Localization of macrophage migration inhibitory factor (MIF) to secretory granules within the corticotrophic and thyrotrophic cells of the pituitary gland. *Mol Med* 1:781-788.
35. Flieger, O., A. Engling, R. Bucala, H. Lue, W. Nickel, and J. Bernhagen. 2003. Regulated secretion of macrophage migration inhibitory factor is mediated by a non-classical pathway involving an ABC transporter. *FEBS Lett* 551:78-86.
36. Merk, M., J. Baugh, S. Zierow, L. Leng, U. Pal, S. J. Lee, A. D. Ebert, Y. Mizue, J. O. Trent, R. Mitchell, W. Nickel, P. B. Kavathas, J. Bernhagen, and R. Bucala. 2009. The Golgi-associated protein p115 mediates the secretion of macrophage migration inhibitory factor. *J Immunol* 182:6896-6906.
37. Mitchell, R. A., C. N. Metz, T. Peng, and R. Bucala. 1999. Sustained mitogen-activated protein kinase (MAPK) and cytoplasmic phospholipase A2 activation by macrophage migration inhibitory factor (MIF). Regulatory role in cell proliferation and glucocorticoid action. *J Biol Chem* 274:18100-18106.
38. Shi, X., L. Leng, T. Wang, W. Wang, X. Du, J. Li, C. McDonald, Z. Chen, J. W. Murphy, E. Lolis, P. Noble, W. Knudson, and R. Bucala. 2006. CD44 is the signaling component of the macrophage migration inhibitory factor-CD74 receptor complex. *Immunity* 25:595-606.
39. Lesley, J., R. Hyman, and P. W. Kincade. 1993. CD44 and its interaction with extracellular matrix. *Adv Immunol* 54:271-335.
40. Tarnowski, M., K. Grymula, R. Liu, J. Tarnowska, J. Drukala, J. Ratajczak, R. A. Mitchell, M. Z. Ratajczak, and M. Kucia. Macrophage migration inhibitory factor is secreted by rhabdomyosarcoma cells, modulates tumor metastasis by

binding to CXCR4 and CXCR7 receptors and inhibits recruitment of cancer-associated fibroblasts. *Mol Cancer Res* 8:1328-1343.
41. Lue, H., A. Kapurniotu, G. Fingerle-Rowson, T. Roger, L. Leng, M. Thiele, T. Calandra, R. Bucala, and J. Bernhagen. 2006. Rapid and transient activation of the ERK MAPK signalling pathway by macrophage migration inhibitory factor (MIF) and dependence on JAB1/CSN5 and Src kinase activity. *Cell Signal* 18:688-703.
42. Exton, J. H. 1994. Phosphatidylcholine breakdown and signal transduction. *Biochim Biophys Acta* 1212:26-42.
43. Murakami, M., Y. Nakatani, G. Atsumi, K. Inoue, and I. Kudo. 1997. Regulatory functions of phospholipase A2. *Crit Rev Immunol* 17:225-283.
44. Seibert, K., and J. L. Masferrer. 1994. Role of inducible cyclooxygenase (COX-2) in inflammation. *Receptor* 4:17-23.
45. Goppelt-Struebe, M., and W. Rehfeldt. 1992. Glucocorticoids inhibit TNF alpha-induced cytosolic phospholipase A2 activity. *Biochim Biophys Acta* 1127:163-167.
46. Vojtek, A. B., and C. J. Der. 1998. Increasing complexity of the Ras signaling pathway. *J Biol Chem* 273:19925-19928.
47. Robinson, M. J., and M. H. Cobb. 1997. Mitogen-activated protein kinase pathways. *Curr Opin Cell Biol* 9:180-186.
48. Howe, A. K., and R. L. Juliano. 1998. Distinct mechanisms mediate the initial and sustained phases of integrin-mediated activation of the Raf/MEK/mitogen-activated protein kinase cascade. *J Biol Chem* 273:27268-27274.
49. Eliceiri, B. P., R. Klemke, S. Stromblad, and D. A. Cheresh. 1998. Integrin alphavbeta3 requirement for sustained mitogen-activated protein kinase activity during angiogenesis. *J Cell Biol* 140:1255-1263.
50. Roovers, K., G. Davey, X. Zhu, M. E. Bottazzi, and R. K. Assoian. 1999. Alpha5beta1 integrin controls cyclin D1 expression by sustaining mitogen-activated protein kinase activity in growth factor-treated cells. *Mol Biol Cell* 10:3197-3204.
51. Roger, T., A. L. Chanson, M. Knaup-Reymond, and T. Calandra. 2005. Macrophage migration inhibitory factor promotes innate immune responses by suppressing glucocorticoid-induced expression of mitogen-activated protein kinase phosphatase-1. *Eur J Immunol* 35:3405-3413.
52. Aeberli, D., Y. Yang, A. Mansell, L. Santos, M. Leech, and E. F. Morand. 2006. Endogenous macrophage migration inhibitory factor modulates glucocorticoid sensitivity in macrophages via effects on MAP kinase phosphatase-1 and p38 MAP kinase. *FEBS Lett* 580:974-981.
53. Daun, J. M., and J. G. Cannon. 2000. Macrophage migration inhibitory factor antagonizes hydrocortisone-induced increases in cytosolic IkappaBalpha. *Am J Physiol Regul Integr Comp Physiol* 279:R1043-1049.
54. Medzhitov, R., P. Preston-Hurlburt, and C. A. Janeway, Jr. 1997. A human homologue of the Drosophila Toll protein signals activation of adaptive immunity. *Nature* 388:394-397.
55. Chow, J. C., D. W. Young, D. T. Golenbock, W. J. Christ, and F. Gusovsky. 1999. Toll-like receptor-4 mediates lipopolysaccharide-induced signal transduction. *J Biol Chem* 274:10689-10692.
56. Roger, T., I. Miconnet, A. L. Schiesser, H. Kai, K. Miyake, and T. Calandra. 2005. Critical role for Ets, AP-1 and GATA-like transcription factors in

regulating mouse Toll-like receptor 4 (Tlr4) gene expression. *Biochem J* 387:355-365.
57. Roger, T., J. David, M. P. Glauser, and T. Calandra. 2001. MIF regulates innate immune responses through modulation of Toll-like receptor 4. *Nature* 414:920-924.
58. Barr, P. J., and L. D. Tomei. 1994. Apoptosis and its role in human disease. *Biotechnology (N Y)* 12:487-493.
59. Feng, Q. Z., Y. S. Zhao, and E. Abdelwahid. 2008. The role of Fas in the progression of ischemic heart failure: prohypertrophy or proapoptosis. *Coron Artery Dis* 19:527-534.
60. Kuwano, K., and N. Hara. 2000. Signal transduction pathways of apoptosis and inflammation induced by the tumor necrosis factor receptor family. *Am J Respir Cell Mol Biol* 22:147-149.
61. Messmer, U. K., M. Ankarcrona, P. Nicotera, and B. Brune. 1994. p53 expression in nitric oxide-induced apoptosis. *FEBS Lett* 355:23-26.
62. Hudson, J. D., M. A. Shoaibi, R. Maestro, A. Carnero, G. J. Hannon, and D. H. Beach. 1999. A proinflammatory cytokine inhibits p53 tumor suppressor activity. *J Exp Med* 190:1375-1382.
63. MacMicking, J., Q. W. Xie, and C. Nathan. 1997. Nitric oxide and macrophage function. *Annu Rev Immunol* 15:323-350.
64. Messmer, U. K., E. G. Lapetina, and B. Brune. 1995. Nitric oxide-induced apoptosis in RAW 264.7 macrophages is antagonized by protein kinase C- and protein kinase A-activating compounds. *Mol Pharmacol* 47:757-765.
65. Albina, J. E., S. Cui, R. B. Mateo, and J. S. Reichner. 1993. Nitric oxide-mediated apoptosis in murine peritoneal macrophages. *J Immunol* 150:5080-5085.
66. Sarih, M., V. Souvannavong, and A. Adam. 1993. Nitric oxide synthase induces macrophage death by apoptosis. *Biochem Biophys Res Commun* 191:503-508.
67. Williams, T. E., A. Ayala, and I. H. Chaudry. 1997. Inducible macrophage apoptosis following sepsis is mediated by cysteine protease activation and nitric oxide release. *J Surg Res* 70:113-118.
68. Messmer, U. K., D. M. Reimer, J. C. Reed, and B. Brune. 1996. Nitric oxide induced poly(ADP-ribose) polymerase cleavage in RAW 264.7 macrophage apoptosis is blocked by Bcl-2. *FEBS Lett* 384:162-166.
69. Mitchell, R. A., H. Liao, J. Chesney, G. Fingerle-Rowson, J. Baugh, J. David, and R. Bucala. 2002. Macrophage migration inhibitory factor (MIF) sustains macrophage proinflammatory function by inhibiting p53: regulatory role in the innate immune response. *Proc Natl Acad Sci U S A* 99:345-350.
70. Lue, H., M. Thiele, J. Franz, E. Dahl, S. Speckgens, L. Leng, G. Fingerle-Rowson, R. Bucala, B. Luscher, and J. Bernhagen. 2007. Macrophage migration inhibitory factor (MIF) promotes cell survival by activation of the Akt pathway and role for CSN5/JAB1 in the control of autocrine MIF activity. *Oncogene* 26:5046-5059.
71. Datta, S. R., A. M. Ranger, M. Z. Lin, J. F. Sturgill, Y. C. Ma, C. W. Cowan, P. Dikkes, S. J. Korsmeyer, and M. E. Greenberg. 2002. Survival factor-mediated BAD phosphorylation raises the mitochondrial threshold for apoptosis. *Dev Cell* 3:631-643.
72. Agarwal, A., K. Das, N. Lerner, S. Sathe, M. Cicek, G. Casey, and N. Sizemore. 2005. The AKT/I kappa B kinase pathway promotes

73. angiogenic/metastatic gene expression in colorectal cancer by activating nuclear factor-kappa B and beta-catenin. *Oncogene* 24:1021-1031.
74. Mantovani, A., P. Allavena, A. Sica, and F. Balkwill. 2008. Cancer-related inflammation. *Nature* 454:436-444.
75. Weber, J. D., D. M. Raben, P. J. Phillips, and J. J. Baldassare. 1997. Sustained activation of extracellular-signal-regulated kinase 1 (ERK1) is required for the continued expression of cyclin D1 in G1 phase. *Biochem J* 326 (Pt 1):61-68.
76. Kleemann, R., A. Hausser, G. Geiger, R. Mischke, A. Burger-Kentischer, O. Flieger, F. J. Johannes, T. Roger, T. Calandra, A. Kapurniotu, M. Grell, D. Finkelmeier, H. Brunner, and J. Bernhagen. 2000. Intracellular action of the cytokine MIF to modulate AP-1 activity and the cell cycle through Jab1. *Nature* 408:211-216.
77. Wiersinga, W. J., and T. van der Poll. [Sepsis: new insights into its pathogenesis and treatment]. *Ned Tijdschr Geneeskd* 154:A1130.
78. Anel, R., and A. Kumar. 2005. Human endotoxemia and human sepsis: limits to the model. *Crit Care* 9:151-152.
79. Levy, M. M., M. P. Fink, J. C. Marshall, E. Abraham, D. Angus, D. Cook, J. Cohen, S. M. Opal, J. L. Vincent, and G. Ramsay. 2003. 2001 SCCM/ESICM/ACCP/ATS/SIS International Sepsis Definitions Conference. *Intensive Care Med* 29:530-538.
80. Anas, A. A., W. J. Wiersinga, A. F. de Vos, and T. van der Poll. Recent insights into the pathogenesis of bacterial sepsis. *Neth J Med* 68:147-152.
81. Bone, R. C., R. A. Balk, F. B. Cerra, R. P. Dellinger, A. M. Fein, W. A. Knaus, R. M. Schein, and W. J. Sibbald. 1992. Definitions for sepsis and organ failure and guidelines for the use of innovative therapies in sepsis. The ACCP/SCCM Consensus Conference Committee. American College of Chest Physicians/Society of Critical Care Medicine. *Chest* 101:1644-1655.
82. Al-Abed, Y., D. Dabideen, B. Aljabari, A. Valster, D. Messmer, M. Ochani, M. Tanovic, K. Ochani, M. Bacher, F. Nicoletti, C. Metz, V. A. Pavlov, E. J. Miller, and K. J. Tracey. 2005. ISO-1 binding to the tautomerase active site of MIF inhibits its pro-inflammatory activity and increases survival in severe sepsis. *J Biol Chem* 280:36541-36544.
83. Calandra, T., B. Echtenacher, D. L. Roy, J. Pugin, C. N. Metz, L. Hultner, D. Heumann, D. Mannel, R. Bucala, and M. P. Glauser. 2000. Protection from septic shock by neutralization of macrophage migration inhibitory factor. *Nat Med* 6:164-170.
84. Matsuda, N., J. Nishihira, Y. Takahashi, O. Kemmotsu, and Y. Hattori. 2006. Role of macrophage migration inhibitory factor in acute lung injury in mice with acute pancreatitis complicated by endotoxemia. *Am J Respir Cell Mol Biol* 35:198-205.
85. Kobayashi, S., J. Nishihira, S. Watanabe, and S. Todo. 1999. Prevention of lethal acute hepatic failure by antimacrophage migration inhibitory factor antibody in mice treated with bacille Calmette-Guerin and lipopolysaccharide. *Hepatology* 29:1752-1759.
86. Garner, L. B., M. S. Willis, D. L. Carlson, J. M. DiMaio, M. D. White, D. J. White, G. A. t. Adams, J. W. Horton, and B. P. Giroir. 2003. Macrophage migration inhibitory factor is a cardiac-derived myocardial depressant factor. *Am J Physiol Heart Circ Physiol* 285:H2500-2509.

86. Pollak, N., T. Sterns, B. Echtenacher, and D. N. Mannel. 2005. Improved resistance to bacterial superinfection in mice by treatment with macrophage migration inhibitory factor. *Infect Immun* 73:6488-6492.
87. Merk, M., S. Zierow, L. Leng, R. Das, X. Du, W. Schulte, J. Fan, H. Lue, Y. Chen, H. Xiong, F. Chagnon, J. Bernhagen, E. Lolis, G. Mor, O. Lesur, and R. Bucala. The D-dopachrome tautomerase (DDT) gene product is a cytokine and functional homolog of macrophage migration inhibitory factor (MIF). *Proc Natl Acad Sci U S A*.
88. Beishuizen, A., L. G. Thijs, C. Haanen, and I. Vermes. 2001. Macrophage migration inhibitory factor and hypothalamo-pituitary-adrenal function during critical illness. *J Clin Endocrinol Metab* 86:2811-2816.
89. Brenner, T., S. Hofer, C. Rosenhagen, J. Steppan, C. Lichtenstern, J. Weitz, T. Bruckner, I. K. Lukic, E. Martin, A. Bierhaus, U. Hoffmann, and M. A. Weigand. Macrophage Migration Inhibitory Factor (MIF) and Manganese Superoxide Dismutase (MnSOD) as Early Predictors for Survival in Patients with Severe Sepsis or Septic Shock. *J Surg Res*.
90. Lai, K. N., J. C. Leung, C. N. Metz, F. M. Lai, R. Bucala, and H. Y. Lan. 2003. Role for macrophage migration inhibitory factor in acute respiratory distress syndrome. *J Pathol* 199:496-508.
91. Magalhaes, E. S., D. S. Mourao-Sa, A. Vieira-de-Abreu, R. T. Figueiredo, A. L. Pires, F. A. Farias-Filho, B. P. Fonseca, J. P. Viola, C. Metz, M. A. Martins, H. C. Castro-Faria-Neto, P. T. Bozza, and M. T. Bozza. 2007. Macrophage migration inhibitory factor is essential for allergic asthma but not for Th2 differentiation. *Eur J Immunol* 37:1097-1106.
92. Mikulowska, A., C. N. Metz, R. Bucala, and R. Holmdahl. 1997. Macrophage migration inhibitory factor is involved in the pathogenesis of collagen type II-induced arthritis in mice. *J Immunol* 158:5514-5517.
93. Leech, M., C. Metz, L. Santos, T. Peng, S. R. Holdsworth, R. Bucala, and E. F. Morand. 1998. Involvement of macrophage migration inhibitory factor in the evolution of rat adjuvant arthritis. *Arthritis Rheum* 41:910-917.
94. Santos, L., P. Hall, C. Metz, R. Bucala, and E. F. Morand. 2001. Role of macrophage migration inhibitory factor (MIF) in murine antigen-induced arthritis: interaction with glucocorticoids. *Clin Exp Immunol* 123:309-314.
95. Leech, M., C. Metz, P. Hall, P. Hutchinson, K. Gianis, M. Smith, H. Weedon, S. R. Holdsworth, R. Bucala, and E. F. Morand. 1999. Macrophage migration inhibitory factor in rheumatoid arthritis: evidence of proinflammatory function and regulation by glucocorticoids. *Arthritis Rheum* 42:1601-1608.
96. Onodera, S., H. Tanji, K. Suzuki, K. Kaneda, Y. Mizue, A. Sagawa, and J. Nishihira. 1999. High expression of macrophage migration inhibitory factor in the synovial tissues of rheumatoid joints. *Cytokine* 11:163-167.
97. Gregory, J. L., M. T. Leech, J. R. David, Y. H. Yang, A. Dacumos, and M. J. Hickey. 2004. Reduced leukocyte-endothelial cell interactions in the inflamed microcirculation of macrophage migration inhibitory factor-deficient mice. *Arthritis Rheum* 50:3023-3034.
98. Lin, S. G., X. Y. Yu, Y. X. Chen, X. R. Huang, C. Metz, R. Bucala, C. P. Lau, and H. Y. Lan. 2000. De novo expression of macrophage migration inhibitory factor in atherogenesis in rabbits. *Circ Res* 87:1202-1208.
99. Burger-Kentischer, A., H. Goebel, R. Seiler, G. Fraedrich, H. E. Schaefer, S. Dimmeler, R. Kleemann, J. Bernhagen, and C. Ihling. 2002. Expression of

macrophage migration inhibitory factor in different stages of human atherosclerosis. *Circulation* 105:1561-1566.
100. Burger-Kentischer, A., H. Gobel, R. Kleemann, A. Zernecke, R. Bucala, L. Leng, D. Finkelmeier, G. Geiger, H. E. Schaefer, A. Schober, C. Weber, H. Brunner, H. Rutten, C. Ihling, and J. Bernhagen. 2006. Reduction of the aortic inflammatory response in spontaneous atherosclerosis by blockade of macrophage migration inhibitory factor (MIF). *Atherosclerosis* 184:28-38.
101. Amin, M. A., C. S. Haas, K. Zhu, P. J. Mansfield, M. J. Kim, N. P. Lackowski, and A. E. Koch. 2006. Migration inhibitory factor up-regulates vascular cell adhesion molecule-1 and intercellular adhesion molecule-1 via Src, PI3 kinase, and NFkappaB. *Blood* 107:2252-2261.
102. Morand, E. F., M. Leech, and J. Bernhagen. 2006. MIF: a new cytokine link between rheumatoid arthritis and atherosclerosis. *Nat Rev Drug Discov* 5:399-410.
103. Libby, P. 2002. Inflammation in atherosclerosis. *Nature* 420:868-874.
104. Ishizaka, K., Y. Ishii, T. Nakano, and K. Sugie. 2000. Biochemical basis of antigen-specific suppressor T cell factors: controversies and possible answers. *Adv Immunol* 74:1-60.
105. Wistow, G. J., M. P. Shaughnessy, D. C. Lee, J. Hodin, and P. S. Zelenka. 1993. A macrophage migration inhibitory factor is expressed in the differentiating cells of the eye lens. *Proc Natl Acad Sci U S A* 90:1272-1275.
106. Sato, A., T. S. Uinuk-ool, N. Kuroda, W. E. Mayer, N. Takezaki, R. Dongak, F. Figueroa, M. D. Cooper, and J. Klein. 2003. Macrophage migration inhibitory factor (MIF) of jawed and jawless fishes: implications for its evolutionary origin. *Dev Comp Immunol* 27:401-412.
107. Jaworski, D. C., A. Jasinskas, C. N. Metz, R. Bucala, and A. G. Barbour. 2001. Identification and characterization of a homologue of the pro-inflammatory cytokine Macrophage Migration Inhibitory Factor in the tick, Amblyomma americanum. *Insect Mol Biol* 10:323-331.
108. Pastrana, D. V., N. Raghavan, P. FitzGerald, S. W. Eisinger, C. Metz, R. Bucala, R. P. Schleimer, C. Bickel, and A. L. Scott. 1998. Filarial nematode parasites secrete a homologue of the human cytokine macrophage migration inhibitory factor. *Infect Immun* 66:5955-5963.
109. Guiliano, D. B., N. Hall, S. J. Jones, L. N. Clark, C. H. Corton, B. G. Barrell, and M. L. Blaxter. 2002. Conservation of long-range synteny and microsynteny between the genomes of two distantly related nematodes. *Genome Biol* 3:RESEARCH0057.
110. Sun, H. W., J. Bernhagen, R. Bucala, and E. Lolis. 1996. Crystal structure at 2.6-A resolution of human macrophage migration inhibitory factor. *Proc Natl Acad Sci U S A* 93:5191-5196.
111. Suzuki, M., H. Sugimoto, A. Nakagawa, I. Tanaka, J. Nishihira, and M. Sakai. 1996. Crystal structure of the macrophage migration inhibitory factor from rat liver. *Nat Struct Biol* 3:259-266.
112. Sugimoto, H., M. Suzuki, A. Nakagawa, I. Tanaka, and J. Nishihira. 1996. Crystal structure of macrophage migration inhibitory factor from human lymphocyte at 2.1 A resolution. *FEBS Lett* 389:145-148.
113. Muhlhahn, P., J. Bernhagen, M. Czisch, J. Georgescu, C. Renner, A. Ross, R. Bucala, and T. A. Holak. 1996. NMR characterization of structure, backbone

dynamics, and glutathione binding of the human macrophage migration inhibitory factor (MIF). *Protein Sci* 5:2095-2103.
114. Mischke, R., R. Kleemann, H. Brunner, and J. Bernhagen. 1998. Cross-linking and mutational analysis of the oligomerization state of the cytokine macrophage migration inhibitory factor (MIF). *FEBS Lett* 427:85-90.
115. Subramanya, H. S., D. I. Roper, Z. Dauter, E. J. Dodson, G. J. Davies, K. S. Wilson, and D. B. Wigley. 1996. Enzymatic ketonization of 2-hydroxymuconate: specificity and mechanism investigated by the crystal structures of two isomerases. *Biochemistry* 35:792-802.
116. Merk, M. 2008. Molecular Mechanisms of the Unconventional Secretion of Macrophage Migration Inhibitory Factor (MIF). In *Institut für Biochemie, Abteilung Biochemie und Molekulare Zellbiologie*. RWTH Aachen und Yale University School of Medicine.
117. Kleemann, R., A. Kapurniotu, R. W. Frank, A. Gessner, R. Mischke, O. Flieger, S. Juttner, H. Brunner, and J. Bernhagen. 1998. Disulfide analysis reveals a role for macrophage migration inhibitory factor (MIF) as thiol-protein oxidoreductase. *J Mol Biol* 280:85-102.
118. Kleemann, R., R. Mischke, A. Kapurniotu, H. Brunner, and J. Bernhagen. 1998. Specific reduction of insulin disulfides by macrophage migration inhibitory factor (MIF) with glutathione and dihydrolipoamide: potential role in cellular redox processes. *FEBS Lett* 430:191-196.
119. Kleemann, R., H. Rorsman, E. Rosengren, R. Mischke, N. T. Mai, and J. Bernhagen. 2000. Dissection of the enzymatic and immunologic functions of macrophage migration inhibitory factor. Full immunologic activity of N-terminally truncated mutants. *Eur J Biochem* 267:7183-7193.
120. Burger-Kentischer, A., D. Finkelmeier, M. Thiele, J. Schmucker, G. Geiger, G. E. Tovar, and J. Bernhagen. 2005. Binding of JAB1/CSN5 to MIF is mediated by the MPN domain but is independent of the JAMM motif. *FEBS Lett* 579:1693-1701.
121. Swope, M. D., and E. Lolis. 1999. Macrophage migration inhibitory factor: cytokine, hormone, or enzyme? *Reviews of physiology, biochemistry and pharmacology* 139:1-32.
122. Lubetsky, J. B., M. Swope, C. Dealwis, P. Blake, and E. Lolis. 1999. Pro-1 of macrophage migration inhibitory factor functions as a catalytic base in the phenylpyruvate tautomerase activity. *Biochemistry* 38:7346-7354.
123. Lubetsky, J. B., A. Dios, J. Han, B. Aljabari, B. Ruzsicska, R. Mitchell, E. Lolis, and Y. Al-Abed. 2002. The tautomerase active site of macrophage migration inhibitory factor is a potential target for discovery of novel anti-inflammatory agents. *The Journal of biological chemistry* 277:24976-24982.
124. Swope, M., H. W. Sun, P. R. Blake, and E. Lolis. 1998. Direct link between cytokine activity and a catalytic site for macrophage migration inhibitory factor. *EMBO J* 17:3534-3541.
125. Onodera, S., K. Kaneda, Y. Mizue, Y. Koyama, M. Fujinaga, and J. Nishihira. 2000. Macrophage migration inhibitory factor up-regulates expression of matrix metalloproteinases in synovial fibroblasts of rheumatoid arthritis. *J Biol Chem* 275:444-450.
126. Senter, P. D., Y. Al-Abed, C. N. Metz, F. Benigni, R. A. Mitchell, J. Chesney, J. Han, C. G. Gartner, S. D. Nelson, G. J. Todaro, and R. Bucala. 2002. Inhibition of macrophage migration inhibitory factor (MIF) tautomerase and

biological activities by acetaminophen metabolites. *Proc Natl Acad Sci U S A* 99:144-149.

127. Winner, M., J. Meier, S. Zierow, B. E. Rendon, G. V. Crichlow, R. Riggs, R. Bucala, L. Leng, N. Smith, E. Lolis, J. O. Trent, and R. A. Mitchell. 2008. A novel, macrophage migration inhibitory factor suicide substrate inhibits motility and growth of lung cancer cells. *Cancer research* 68:7253-7257.

128. Al-Abed, Y., C. N. Metz, K. F. Cheng, B. Aljabari, S. Vanpatten, S. Blau, H. Lee, M. Ochani, V. A. Pavlov, T. Coleman, N. Meurice, K. J. Tracey, and E. J. Miller. Thyroxine is a potential endogenous antagonist of macrophage migration inhibitory factor (MIF) activity. *Proc Natl Acad Sci U S A*.

129. Aroca, P., J. C. Garcia-Borron, F. Solano, and J. A. Lozano. 1990. Regulation of mammalian melanogenesis. I: Partial purification and characterization of a dopachrome converting factor: dopachrome tautomerase. *Biochim Biophys Acta* 1035:266-275.

130. Tsukamoto, K., I. J. Jackson, K. Urabe, P. M. Montague, and V. J. Hearing. 1992. A second tyrosinase-related protein, TRP-2, is a melanogenic enzyme termed DOPAchrome tautomerase. *EMBO J* 11:519-526.

131. Winder, A. J., A. Wittbjer, E. Rosengren, and H. Rorsman. 1993. The mouse brown (b) locus protein has dopachrome tautomerase activity and is located in lysosomes in transfected fibroblasts. *J Cell Sci* 106 (Pt 1):153-166.

132. Odh, G., A. Hindemith, A. M. Rosengren, E. Rosengren, and H. Rorsman. 1993. Isolation of a new tautomerase monitored by the conversion of D-dopachrome to 5,6-dihydroxyindole. *Biochem Biophys Res Commun* 197:619-624.

133. Bjork, P., P. Aman, A. Hindemith, G. Odh, L. Jacobsson, E. Rosengren, and H. Rorsman. 1996. A new enzyme activity in human blood cells and isolation of the responsible protein (D-dopachrome tautomerase) from erythrocytes. *Eur J Haematol* 57:254-256.

134. Yokoyama, K., K. Yasumoto, H. Suzuki, and S. Shibahara. 1994. Cloning of the human DOPAchrome tautomerase/tyrosinase-related protein 2 gene and identification of two regulatory regions required for its pigment cell-specific expression. *J Biol Chem* 269:27080-27087.

135. Sugimoto, H., M. Taniguchi, A. Nakagawa, I. Tanaka, M. Suzuki, and J. Nishihira. 1999. Crystal structure of human D-dopachrome tautomerase, a homologue of macrophage migration inhibitory factor, at 1.54 A resolution. *Biochemistry* 38:3268-3279.

136. Rosengren, E., R. Bucala, P. Aman, L. Jacobsson, G. Odh, C. N. Metz, and H. Rorsman. 1996. The immunoregulatory mediator macrophage migration inhibitory factor (MIF) catalyzes a tautomerization reaction. *Mol Med* 2:143-149.

137. Rosengren, E., P. Aman, S. Thelin, C. Hansson, S. Ahlfors, P. Bjork, L. Jacobsson, and H. Rorsman. 1997. The macrophage migration inhibitory factor MIF is a phenylpyruvate tautomerase. *FEBS Lett* 417:85-88.

138. Nishihira, J., M. Fujinaga, T. Kuriyama, M. Suzuki, H. Sugimoto, A. Nakagawa, I. Tanaka, and M. Sakai. 1998. Molecular cloning of human D-dopachrome tautomerase cDNA: N-terminal proline is essential for enzyme activation. *Biochem Biophys Res Commun* 243:538-544.

139. Sonesson, B., E. Rosengren, A. S. Hansson, and C. Hansson. 2003. UVB-induced inflammation gives increased d-dopachrome tautomerase activity in

blister fluid which correlates with macrophage migration inhibitory factor. *Exp Dermatol* 12:278-282.
140. Coleman, A. M., B. E. Rendon, M. Zhao, M. W. Qian, R. Bucala, D. Xin, and R. A. Mitchell. 2008. Cooperative regulation of non-small cell lung carcinoma angiogenic potential by macrophage migration inhibitory factor and its homolog, D-dopachrome tautomerase. *J Immunol* 181:2330-2337.
141. Xin, D., B. E. Rendon, M. Zhao, M. Winner, A. McGhee Coleman, and R. A. Mitchell. The MIF homologue D-dopachrome tautomerase promotes COX-2 expression through beta-catenin-dependent and -independent mechanisms. *Mol Cancer Res* 8:1601-1609.
142. Hiyoshi, M., H. Konishi, H. Uemura, H. Matsuzaki, H. Tsukamoto, R. Sugimoto, H. Takeda, S. Dakeshita, A. Kitayama, H. Takami, F. Sawachika, H. Kido, and K. Arisawa. 2009. D-Dopachrome tautomerase is a candidate for key proteins to protect the rat liver damaged by carbon tetrachloride. *Toxicology* 255:6-14.
143. Smyth, R., C. S. Lane, R. Ashiq, J. A. Turton, C. J. Clarke, T. O. Dare, M. J. York, W. Griffiths, and M. R. Munday. 2009. Proteomic investigation of urinary markers of carbon-tetrachloride-induced hepatic fibrosis in the Hanover Wistar rat. *Cell Biol Toxicol* 25:499-512.
144. Bradford, M. M. 1976. A rapid and sensitive method for the quantitation of microgram quantities of protein utilizing the principle of protein-dye binding. *Anal Biochem* 72:248-254.
145. Liao, H., R. Bucala, and R. A. Mitchell. 2003. Adhesion-dependent signaling by macrophage migration inhibitory factor (MIF). *J Biol Chem* 278:76-81.
146. Zhang, M., P. Aman, A. Grubb, I. Panagopoulos, A. Hindemith, E. Rosengren, and H. Rorsman. 1995. Cloning and sequencing of a cDNA encoding rat D-dopachrome tautomerase. *FEBS Lett* 373:203-206.
147. Gore, Y., D. Starlets, N. Maharshak, S. Becker-Herman, U. Kaneyuki, L. Leng, R. Bucala, and I. Shachar. 2008. Macrophage migration inhibitory factor induces B cell survival by activation of a CD74-CD44 receptor complex. *J Biol Chem* 283:2784-2792.
148. Holton, T. A., and M. W. Graham. 1991. A simple and efficient method for direct cloning of PCR products using ddT-tailed vectors. *Nucleic Acids Res* 19:1156.
149. Dalby, B., S. Cates, A. Harris, E. C. Ohki, M. L. Tilkins, P. J. Price, and V. C. Ciccarone. 2004. Advanced transfection with Lipofectamine 2000 reagent: primary neurons, siRNA, and high-throughput applications. *Methods* 33:95-103.
150. Lakshmipathy, U., S. Buckley, and C. Verfaillie. 2007. Gene transfer via nucleofection into adult and embryonic stem cells. *Methods Mol Biol* 407:115-126.
151. Miller, E. J., J. Li, L. Leng, C. McDonald, T. Atsumi, R. Bucala, and L. H. Young. 2008. Macrophage migration inhibitory factor stimulates AMP-activated protein kinase in the ischaemic heart. *Nature* 451:578-582.
152. Bendrat, K., Y. Al-Abed, D. J. Callaway, T. Peng, T. Calandra, C. N. Metz, and R. Bucala. 1997. Biochemical and mutational investigations of the enzymatic activity of macrophage migration inhibitory factor. *Biochemistry* 36:15356-15362.

153. Stamps, S. L., M. C. Fitzgerald, and C. P. Whitman. 1998. Characterization of the role of the amino-terminal proline in the enzymatic activity catalyzed by macrophage migration inhibitory factor. *Biochemistry* 37:10195-10202.
154. Grieb, G., M. Merk, J. Bernhagen, and R. Bucala. Macrophage migration inhibitory factor (MIF): a promising biomarker. *Drug News Perspect* 23:257-264.

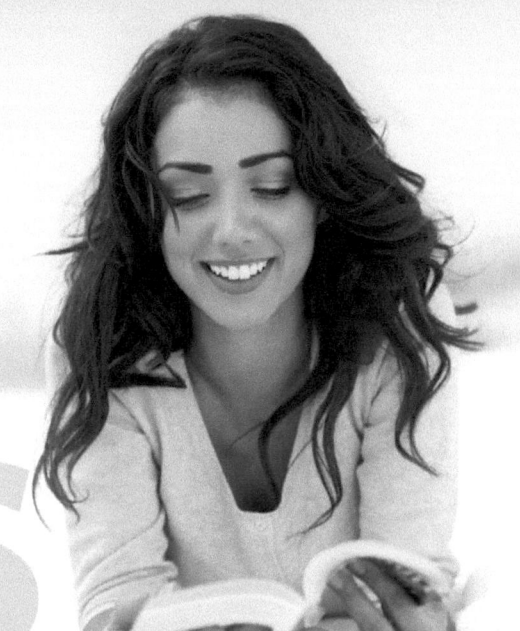

i want morebooks!

Buy your books fast and straightforward online - at one of world's fastest growing online book stores! Environmentally sound due to Print-on-Demand technologies.

Buy your books online at

www.get-morebooks.com

Kaufen Sie Ihre Bücher schnell und unkompliziert online – auf einer der am schnellsten wachsenden Buchhandelsplattformen weltweit! Dank Print-On-Demand umwelt- und ressourcenschonend produziert.

Bücher schneller online kaufen

www.morebooks.de

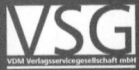

VDM Verlagsservicegesellschaft mbH
Heinrich-Böcking-Str. 6-8
D - 66121 Saarbrücken

Telefon: +49 681 3720 174
Telefax: +49 681 3720 1749

info@vdm-vsg.de
www.vdm-vsg.de

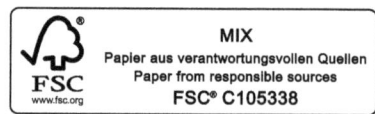

Printed by Books on Demand GmbH, Norderstedt / Germany